TMJ
THE JAW CONNECTION

TMJ
THE JAW CONNECTION
THE OVERLOOKED DIAGNOSIS
A Self-Care Guide to Diagnosing and
Managing this Hidden Ailment

Greg Goddard, D.D.S

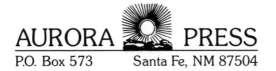

AURORA PRESS
P.O. Box 573   Santa Fe, NM 87504

ISBN: 0-943358-35-3
LC #91-75870

A publication of
Aurora Press
P O Box 573
Santa Fe, NM 87504
USA

This book is set in 12 point Souvenir type

Photographs by *Mikkel Aaland*
Illustrations by *Jose Dumas*

Printed in the United States of America

2P93

CONTENTS

Contents

ACKNOWLEDGEMENTS

The writing of this book took place because of a need that I saw, and a service that patients requested. I would like to thank those patients who, in discussing how to manage their problems, gave me feedback and knowledge of what things were important to do, and what things were not. I would especially like to thank the Native American Indian community, which I have had the privilege to serve these past fifteen years. I also would like to thank my employer, the Urban Indian Health Board.

I must also thank my teacher of over twenty years ago, David Downton, F.D.S.R.C.S., of the Royal Free Hospital in London, England. He taught me the basic principles of orthopedics, of treating TMJ the same as one would treat any joint in the body. I must also thank all the researchers in the United States who twenty years ago believed that the problems with TMJ were largely caused by the teeth. They have opened their eyes to the scientific evidence that supports treating TMJ like other joints in the body.

Special thanks goes to Patricia Rudd, R.P.T., who encouraged and supported my original idea of a book for patients. Her ability to see clearly through so much of the contradictory research helped and encouraged me to clarify my viewpoint. Her help in reading the manuscript and offering criticism and suggestions was very much appreciated.

Michael Griffiths, D.D.S., was instrumental in shaping the psychological aspects of TMJ problems. Michael Clarke, D.D.S., provided good suggestions and criticisms, as well as encouragement. Jeffrey Wong, D.D.S. helped clarify the role of orthodontics.

And I would like to thank the many others who read my manuscript and gave me feedback, and to the many others who so ably helped with editing, especially Michael Castleman, Barbara Ramsey, MD, and Barbara Armentrout.

I would also like to thank Mikkel Aaland for his photography. My daughter Vari was also very helpful with her support, and in helping with the artwork. My daughter Heather also is greatly appreciated for her modeling skills. Angela Casey and Gioana were also great models. Jose Dumas did the excellent illustrations that helped make this book. Thanks also goes to Helen Friedman for the typing and helpful suggestions.

I must give special thanks to my wife Miguelina, who supported me through all the ups and downs that went along with the year and a half that it took to write this book. And my daughter of five years, Camila, was an inspiration with her ever optimistic outlook on life.

FOREWORD
by Patricia Rudd, P.T.

A temporomandibular joint (jaw) problem used to mean that a patient was headed for numerous conflicting professional opinions and treatment plans. Fortunately in recent years, the treatment has become more standardized. It is managed more like other orthopedic problems. One big difference between say a knee problem and a jaw problem is that the jaw problem is an orthopedic condition primarily managed by a dental professional instead of an orthopedist. Initially, this was confusing not only to patients but to insurance companies. The question was, "Is this a dental or a medical problem?" We now recognize that this is indeed a medical problem!

Since there has been so much misinformation in the past about what a TMJ (jaw) problem is, and what treatment is appropriate, it has become imperative for the patient and practitioners to be knowledgeable about their care. This means that patient and professional education is critical. Dr. Goddard's TMJ book is a comprehensive resource. He does an excellent job describing what medical signs and symptoms to look for, what professionals treat these problems, what the rationale for treatment is, and what can be done to participate in this sometimes complex process.

The need for patient participation cannot be emphasized enough. Everyday as a physical therapist, I witness the benefits of patients who are active participants in their care. These patients manage their jaw problem the best. They not only understand their jaw problem and treatment plan, but they understand the importance of their self-care program. The self-care program is one of the keys to managing this problem not only now, but for a lifetime. Dr. Goddard's chapter on self-care tips is one to be read and re-read. He familiarizes the patient with many of the current self-care treatments. He explains what to do, and how this helps decrease jaw pain and restore more normal jaw function.

This handbook is a must for any patient experiencing jaw problems. It is not only a valuable reference on the current philosophy in jaw treatment, but it is written in terms that are easy for patients to read and understand. Professionals should also read this book, have it in their waiting rooms, and recommend it to their patients.

Patricia Rudd, P.T., maintains a private practice in San Francisco, California, with an emphasis on the treatment of temporomandibular disorders.

INTRODUCTION

In the twenty-two years I have been practicing dentistry, I have seen tremendous progress in the understanding of TMJ (temporomandibular joint) disorders. In the past, the majority of problems were thought to be caused by bad bites, but today there's much greater understanding of the role of muscles, joints, stress, tension, and accidents on the TMJ.

Another tremendous change has been the demise of the idea that the doctor does everything for the patient and the patient obeys the doctor. Patients today want a say in their care. In everything from breast cancer treatments to treatment of the TMJ, patients want to be educated, they want to understand their problems, and they want to know the alternative treatments and have a say in what their treatment is all about.

All the progress in scientific understanding about treating TMJ disorders has been written up in journals and textbooks for doctors and dentists. This information now needs to be delivered to the patients. I have found in my practice of dentistry that whenever I can break down the scientific, technical language and translate it into a simple form that patients can understand, they have been able to grasp that knowledge and use it to help in the treatment and management of their problems.

I feel that this kind of patient education is necessary for TMJ disorders. TMJ disorders have been sensationalized, they have been featured in women's magazines, they have been discussed on television programs, TV personalities have talked about them, but sensationalism does not necessarily lead to understanding. What leads to understanding is a concise, simple presentation of the facts in a way that patients can understand, and that is what I attempt to do in this book.

Medicine has used patient education in many other health spheres from alcohol and tobacco use to back problems. The specialized field of health education has been developed to teach people how to deal with their health problems. Because many health problems are not amenable to treatment by medicines and doctors and surgery alone, patients need to understand the disorder or the disease and participate in the treatment in order for it to be a success.

TMJ disorders are one of those areas of health treatment that can be greatly improved by participation and understanding of the patient. I hope that this book will help educate patients, who will then demand more say in their care and, as a result, raise the quality of care they receive.

Disclaimer

The names of all people mentioned in this book have been changed to protect their privacy. The case histories are based on actual cases, but names and details have been changed.

This book tries to provide an understanding of TMJ problems and what one can do to help manage them. It is not meant to take the place of professional advice, and it is not recommended that this book be used for self-diagnosis. A competent medical professional should be consulted for diagnosis and medical advice, as head and neck pain can be an indication of serious conditions.

CHAPTER 1

THE CONTROVERSIAL TMJ

A few years ago the rumor was going around that Burt Reynolds had AIDS: he looked ill, he wasn't able to work, he had lost a lot of weight. It turned out that he had a TMJ disorder as a result of getting hit in the jaw while filming *City Heat*. In a newspaper interview (*San Francisco Chronicle*, May 24, 1987), he described his symptoms: "When your jaw, your bite, goes off, your equilibrium goes off too. You're in a kind of brain pain that comes up and whips your eyeballs out. Then the nausea starts. It's like being seasick all the time. You throw up, can't lie down, can't take any light. If the phone rang, I'd fall on the floor with a pillow over my head because of the pain. I had tubes in my ears and I didn't eat — just drank soup. I kept getting thinner and thinner. It was scary." He saw thirteen dentists before he found one that could alleviate the pain.

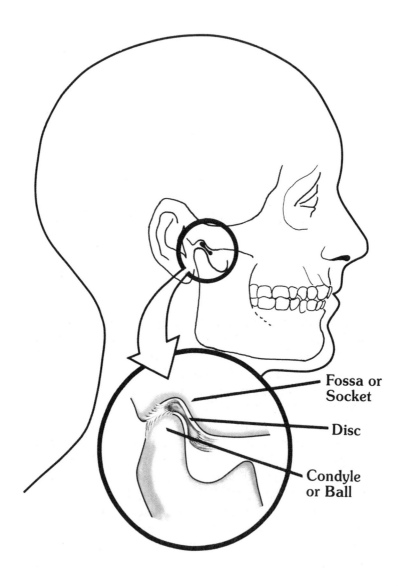

Normal TMJ With Disc As A Cushion

Fossa or
Socket

Disc

Condyle
or Ball

What Is the TMJ?

TMJ is the abbreviation for temporomandibular joint (also called the cranio-mandibular joint). A joint is where two bones join together. You have two TMJs — one in front of each ear connected to the horseshoe-shaped jawbone that has your lower teeth in it. The TMJ is a ball-and-socket joint. The jaw has rounded ends that fit into a socket and slide on a disc, or pad, as your mouth opens for chewing, biting, eating, talking, yawning, kissing, or making various facial expressions. Your lower teeth need to mesh in a very precise way with your upper teeth when your jawbone opens and closes. Your TMJ can give you problems for many different reasons, and we'll discuss each of them in Chapter 5.

The TMJ Controversies

Burt Reynolds' story illustrates the two kinds of controversy surrounding TMJ: its symptoms can be confused with a lot of other illnesses, and its cure is far from agreed upon. The reason for the difficulty diagnosing TMJ disorders is that pain in one part of your body can be referred to other parts through the connecting nerves and muscles. The reason why the treatment of TMJ disorders is controversial is that the causes are still not fully understood.

The controversy over treating TMJ disorders was evident at a workshop of the American Dental Association in late 1989. A lawsuit had been filed to stop eleven experts from discussing the treatment and diagnosis of TMJ disorders, but it was not successful, and 700 dentists signed up for this workshop that had originally been scheduled for a 225-person auditorium.

The main source of conflict over TMJ disorders in the

dental profession is the role of a bad bite, or malocclusion. A large segment of the dental profession believes that bad bites cause TMJ disorders, and therefore the treatment is bite correction at prices that can range from a few thousand dollars up to $15,000 or $20,000 if every tooth has to be capped. The accumulated scientific evidence doesn't substantiate this expensive treatment, however. It favors a more conservative and cost-efficient therapy that includes a soft diet, use of heat and ice, medications, stress management, and splint therapy. For a small percentage of the cases, surgery may be recommended.

The experts at the ADA workshop reported that a survey of the scientific literature showed that TMJ problems may lead to bad bites, but not the reverse, and that TMJ problems may be self-limiting and go away by themselves.[*] This second conclusion was derived from research that showed that most TMJ disorders occur in people between the ages of 24 and 44 and that they rarely occur in people over 65. Because many dentists still believe that malocclusion is the major cause of TMJ disorders and that untreated TMJ problems can lead to permanent degenerative disease, these conclusions were hotly debated at the ADA meeting.

The final word is not yet in, but in the chapters that follow we'll look at various causes of TMJ disorders and the latest scientific evidence about their treatments. This information should help you become an informed consumer of dental treatment and help you to manage your TMJ problem over the long term.

[*] *Cranial Mandibular Disorders, Guidelines for Evaluation, Diagnosis & Management* by American Academy of Cranial Disorders, Charles McNeill DDS. (Quintessence Publishing, 1991).

CHAPTER 2

HOW DO I KNOW IF I HAVE A TMJ DISORDER?

Frank's Toothache

Frank came to my office complaining of a wisdom tooth problem. At least he thought that was the cause of the pain in his jaw that radiated up to his right ear. But when I examined his wisdom tooth, he could open his mouth only about one and a half fingers' width, and I learned that he had had his wisdom teeth removed several years before. He complained that the pain was worse when he opened his mouth. His right temporomandibular joint and both muscles on the right side of the temple and cheek area were very sore to touch. I explained that the problem was not due to his wisdom teeth and asked him if he had hurt his jaw in any way in the past. He remembered that he

7

had been wrestling with a friend the week before and had hit his jaw. It had been sore for a while but he forgot about it until it starting aching a couple of days later. I explained to Frank that he had injured his jaw joint in a way that was similar to an ankle sprain, and that he would need to take care of it in the same way. That would include resting it, which he would need to do by avoiding hard foods and using a soft diet. I instructed him in the use of heat and ice in order to help the jaw joint heal, and showed him some exercises in order to gently stretch and open his mouth. I also told him to take two aspirin every four hours to control the pain and help reduce the swelling in the joint. At the end of a week and a half his pain was completely gone, and he was able to open his jaw normally.

Like Frank, you can have a TMJ disorder without knowing it. Many of the symptoms, such as worn teeth, headaches, neck aches, or earaches, may seem unrelated to your jaw joint, but the TMJ is a complex system, made up of muscles, teeth, nerves, and blood vessels, and the pain will not necessarily be felt in the joint itself. Below are a list of questions that can help you figure out if your pain is due to a TMJ disorder.

1. Do you have headaches frequently?
2. Do your jaws feel tired when you awaken in the morning?
3. Do your jaws ever feel locked?
4. Do you have pain in or above your ears?

5. When you open and close your mouth, does your jaw seem to wiggle or deviate to one side or the other?
6. Are your jaw joints tender when you place your finger over them?
7. Do your teeth ache?
8. Are your teeth wearing down or breaking off?
9. Do you have unexplained pain in your neck, shoulders, or eyes?
10. Do you have difficulty chewing?
11. Does your pain increase after meals or while chewing gum?
12. Does it hurt to move your jaw from side to side?
13. Have you noticed any recent loss of hearing?
14. Do you ever have ringing or hissing in your ears?
15. Do you have unexplained dizziness or feel like you are going to faint?
16. Do you hear or feel a clicking, grating, or popping sound in either of your jaw joints?
17. Do you grind and clench your teeth?
18. Are you unable to open your mouth wide enough to place three fingers between your teeth?
19. Have you ever been involved in an auto accident?
20. Have you ever had a whiplash injury?
21. Have you ever been told to see a psychiatrist or a neurologist because of unexplained head or neck pain?
22. Do you frequently have stiff neck muscles or neck aches?
23. Have you ever had arthritis?
24. Does any family member or relative have arthritis or gout?
25. Have you ever received a severe blow to the head or jaw?

26. Does pain or discomfort from your jaw joint interfere with your work or other activities?
27. Are you under a great deal of stress — job, family, social, school?
28. Do you feel your pain is related to stress?

If you have answered yes to any of the above questions, you may have a TMJ disorder. You can check yourself by performing the five simple tests described later in this chapter. A careful evaluation by a dentist or doctor knowledgeable about this disorder will help you decide whether you have a positive diagnosis. Most patients can be helped, and the majority can be made totally pain free.

How Common Are TMJ Problems?

Studies have shown that between 5 and 7 percent of various populations around the world suffer from TMJ problems. This translates to between 10 and 14 million people in the United States. Most of these studies show that between 60 and 80 percent of the people with TMJ problems are women. The majority of them are between the ages of 30 and 50.

Why are women apparently more susceptible to TMJ problems? First, women may not in fact have more TMJ problems than men. The figures may simply reflect that women in our culture are more likely to seek treatment for pain and that men are more likely to believe they must endure pain.

There are reasons, however, why women may be more prone to TMJ disorders. Women are subject to more stress in our society because they often hold a job and take care of the house and children. Another theory that may explain why more women have TMJ problems is that their bones and joints change during pregnancy. Women go through hormonal changes that soften their bones and allow their joints to stretch in preparation for the baby being born. These hormonal changes in the bones and joints may affect the TMJ. Other studies have shown that women who have excess movement or hypermobility of their hip, elbow, and hand joints are more prone to TMJ problems. Another factor I have seen in my clinical experience is that battered women often suffer from TMJ problems.

To sum all this up, then, women between 30 and 50 may be the most likely to have temporomandibular joint problems, but TMJ disorders can happen for many reasons to people of any age and either sex.

What Tests Can I Do?

1. FEEL YOUR TMJ JOINT
The first test is simply to feel your temporomandibular joint, which is located about one finger's width in front of your ear canal. Press, while slowly opening and closing, and feel if it is painful. Pain indicates something is wrong — either swelling or inflammation. Normal joints should not be painful. Press on your elbow or wrist and move it to compare how a joint should feel.

2. PRESS ON YOUR JAW MUSCLES
The second test is to feel your muscles. Normal muscles should not be painful or sore. Feel, or press, all of your facial and neck muscles for any areas of soreness or tenderness. Try rubbing the muscles on the lower border of your lower jaw. Clench your teeth and feel this muscle

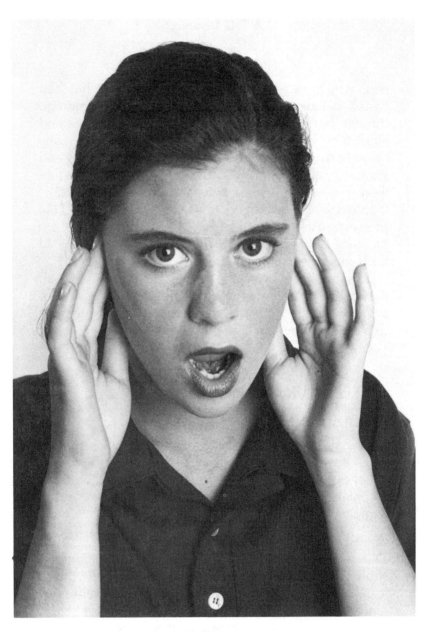

Feeling Your Joints

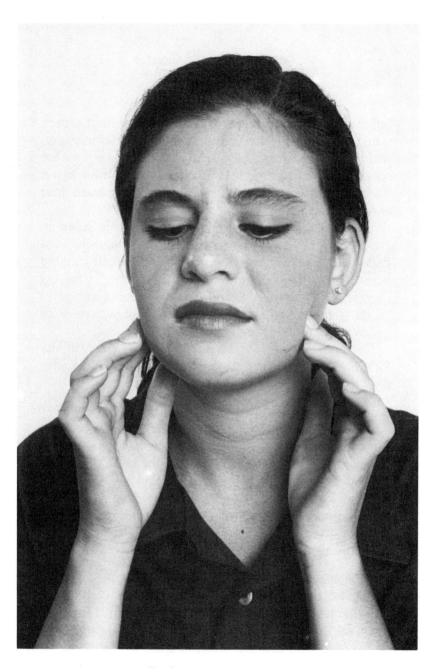

Feeling Your Muscles

bulge. Then press and rub it to see if it is sore. Next, clench your teeth while placing your fingers on your temples and feel the muscle there bulge. Rub and press it to feel for soreness. Feel the muscles in the front of your neck, the back of your neck, and the back of your head and shoulders for soreness or sore spots.

Soreness indicates something is wrong with the muscle. Most of us have experienced sore muscles when we exercise too much. For example, if you go out running when your body is not used to the exercise, your leg muscles will be sore. Similarly, if you do a lot of lifting and you're not used to it, you may find that your back muscles or shoulder muscles are sore.

Muscles also get sore when something is wrong with the joint in order to protect the joint. Muscles also can refer pain to other areas away from the muscle.

3. WATCH YOUR JAW OPEN

The third test for a TMJ problem is to check the movements of your jaw in front of a mirror. First, open your jaw slowly and see if it opens in a straight line or does your jaw deflect to one side or the other? How far can you open your jaw? Can you get at least two and a half fingers between your upper and lower teeth? Does your jaw move the same distance to the right and to the left? If any of these movements are not normal, there could be something wrong with your jaw or your TMJ joint.

4. LISTEN FOR NOISE

Another test is to listen for noises in your joint when you open and close your mouth. Does your joint pop, click, or make grating sounds? Be aware of these sounds.

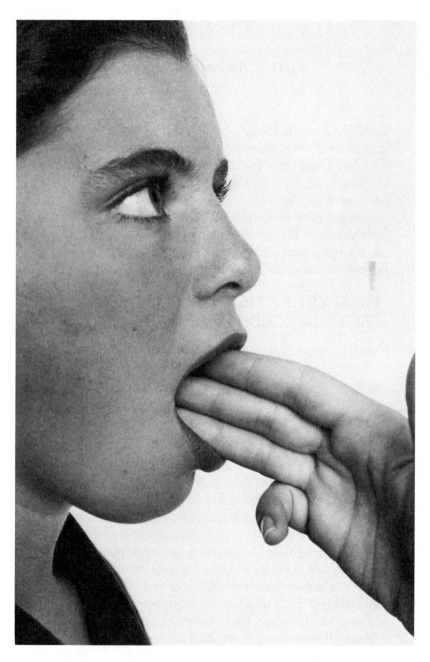

**A Normal Jaw Opening Should Allow Three Fingers
Between Upper And Lower Teeth**

5. CHECK FOR PAIN

You should also observe for pain in your jaw joint or muscles. Does your jaw joint hurt when you chew food? Do you wake up with a sore jaw joint or sore muscles in the morning?

The purpose of these tests is to see if something is not working right. If you have pain or if you cannot properly use your jaw, then you need to have your physician or your dentist examine the problem.

WHAT OTHER MEDICAL PROBLEMS CAN BE CONFUSED WITH TMJ PROBLEMS?

Not all pain in the area of your jaws is caused by problems with the TMJ. Many other problems can mimic the symptoms of TMJ disorders.

HEADACHES

The typical TMJ headache is a pain located on the side of the face in front of the ear with the pain radiating back to the ear, up to the side of the nose and eye, and up onto the temple. Often the TMJ headache is accompanied by dizziness, loss of equilibrium, ringing in the ears, nausea and sensitivity to light. Headaches are very often one of the symptoms of TMJ disorders, but most headache sufferers do not have a TMJ disorder. At most, ten percent of all headaches are from TMJ disorders. There are many different types of headaches, and most of them have nothing to do with TMJ disorders. Headaches affect millions of people regularly, and it is rare to find someone who has never had a headache. Headaches have many different causes.

Migraine

A migraine is a vascular headache characterized by a pre-headache phase that starts about 30 minutes before the actual headache. During this phase there often are visual symptoms ranging from blurriness to partial blindness. Other symptoms may be weakness, dizziness, mental confusion, or even tingling of the feet. Usually these symptoms diminish within 30 minutes and the headache begins, usually on one side of the head. Nausea, vomiting, achiness, and chills often accompany the headache.

Sinus Headache

A sinus headache results from a clogged sinus or an infection of the lining of the sinus. Allergies, most commonly hay fever, can irritate the sinus and cause a headache. Sinus headaches are often associated with colds or flu.

Muscle Contraction Headache

Muscle contraction headache, or tension headache, is the most common type of headache. It is also called a stress headache. It is often described as a tight, viselike band squeezing the head. It usually causes a constant dull ache that can last from hours to days. This type of headache is often associated with TMJ disorders.

Headaches As Symptoms
of Other Medical Conditions

Many medical conditions can cause headaches. Infections, flus, colds, meningitis, head injury, brain tumor, stroke, and high blood pressure are examples. Toothaches can refer pain to the head and are a cause of headaches. Eyestrain, which can be caused by prolonged reading in poor light, can be the source of headaches.

Chemical Headaches

Many chemicals can cause headaches. Probably the best known is the hangover headache caused by alcohol. Other chemicals that can cause headaches are monosodium glutamate (MSG), nitrites (used as food preservatives in bacon and hot dogs), gasoline fumes, paint, paint thinner, glues, and turpentine. Carbon monoxide gas from car exhaust fumes can also cause headaches.

Ear Infection

Probably the disease that most often is confused with TMJ problems is an ear infection. Middle-ear infections are usually seen in young children but occasionally can occur in adults. These infections can cause severe earaches that can be confused with TMJ aches. Usually otitis media, or middle-ear infection, is associated with a fever.

More common in adults is *otitis externa*, often referred to as swimmer's ear. If the ear canal is the site of an infection, the ear and area of the joint become very painful. Pressure on the TMJ can cause pain in this condition. Visual examination by a doctor will usually reveal an infected ear canal.

Sinusitis

Sinusitis can also be confused with temporomandibular joint pain. In sinusitis, the membranes lining the sinuses become inflamed, causing pain that is often felt in the upper teeth and can be referred to the temporomandibular joint.

Temporal Arteritis

Pain from arteries or blood vessels is another source of pain often confused with TMJ pain. One disorder of this type is called temporal arteritis. It is an inflammation of the temporal artery. The patient usually feels a sharp, diffuse pain in front of the ear, and pain can be referred up into the temple area. The pain comes suddenly and lasts for only a short time but returns again and again. Temporal arteritis if left untreated can lead to blindness.

Carotidynia

Another disease of vascular pain is called carotidynia. It causes an intermittent and aching pain over one temporomandibular joint and can radiate up into the temple area and into the ear. In this disease the external carotid artery, which is located in the side of the neck, becomes tender and swollen. Pressure on the artery makes the areas of the face and neck hurt.

Neuralgias

Neuralgias, or nerve pain, can also be confused with temporomandibular joint pain. Even though neuralgias usually cause sharp, severe, stabbing pain, they can at times be confused with temporomandibular joint pain. They can be set off by movement of the jaw, by swallowing, or by touching or moving a specific area. Usually they are differentiated from TMJ pain in that the pain is very severe and lasts for only a very short time.

LYME DISEASE

Bitten by a Tick

Heather complained of pain in her right temporomandibular joint and an inability to open her mouth more than one and a half fingers' width. She also complained of pain in the joints of her knees and shoulders. She had a red rash on her legs that she had said had increased in size over the past week. When further questioned, Heather remembered that she had been bitten by a tick three weeks earlier. She had noticed a red rash around the area where she was bitten. It turned out that Heather had Lyme disease, which is caused by infection from bacteria that are carried in ticks and can cause rashes and pain in various joints of the body. Lyme disease can be treated with antibiotics, as was Heather, and the symptoms promptly disappear.

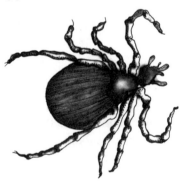

DEER TICK
Carrier of Lyme Disease

Lyme disease is becoming increasingly common in the United States. It is caused by a bacteria carried in ticks. Symptoms include headaches, stiff neck, chills, fever, muscle aches, marked fatigue, nausea, vomiting, skin rashes, and joint pains in various joints of the body, including the temporomandibular joint. A skin rash is seen near the site of the tick bite, and within three or four weeks the rash increases in size. The episodes of the joint pain usually last only about a week at a time. Treatment is with antibiotics, either penicillin or tetracycline. Usually after taking antibiotics for ten to twenty days, the symptoms disappear.

Arthritis

Arthritis, which is an inflammation of a joint, can attack the joints in the neck bones as well as the temporomandibular joint. It can also then cause the muscles that control those joints to become painful in order to protect the joint. There are several types of arthritis.

Osteoarthritis

Osteoarthritis, or degenerative arthritis, is the most common form of arthritis, and it can cause pain on movement of the joints. It is thought that it exists in almost every person in some joint after the age of 25 or 30. It is probably the result of years of wear and tear on the joints. The older one gets, the more evidence there is of osteoarthritis. Trauma to a joint increases the likelihood of osteoarthritis in the future. Osteoarthritis is probably responsible for many of the problems that we associate with aging, because, as people age, their joints become worn and rough and less able to move smoothly and bear up under heavy loads and stress. It is probably one of the reasons that most athletes retire after age 40.

Rheumatoid Arthritis

Rheumatoid arthritis is much rarer than osteoarthritis, but it affects approximately 7 million people in the United States. It usually starts after 40. Rheumatoid arthritis is a type of auto-immune disease. It is a breakdown of the body's immune response system. There is some evidence that it is associated with emotional trauma in some cases. Rheumatoid arthritis usually involves both sides of the body, that is, if it affects the hand and wrist, it's usually both right and left. If it's the knee, it's both knees, and if it's the TMJ, it's usually both of them. It can cause the joints to become red, swollen, and painful. Rheumatoid arthritis usually should be managed by a physician. There are specialists called rheumatologists who specialize in managing this type of arthritis.

Other Types of Arthritis

Osteoarthritis and rheumatoid arthritis are the two major types of arthritis, but there are several other, rarer forms. Gout, juvenile rheumatoid arthritis, ankylosing spondylitis, arthritis from gonorrhea infection, psoriatic arthritis, and Reiters syndrome are other types of arthritis that have been known to affect the TMJ. These types of arthritis are fairly rare, especially in the area of the TMJ. There are many laboratory tests that your physician can perform in order to help diagnose the various types of arthritis.

CHAPTER 3

HOW SHOULD A TMJ DISORDER BE DIAGNOSED?

An accurate diagnosis of your TMJ problem requires a thorough medical and dental evaluation by a trained professional, either a doctor or a dentist.

How should you decide which doctor or dentist to see? First of all, the doctor or dentist must take your complaint seriously. If your problem is serious enough to you to seek out medical help, the person you go to must take your complaints seriously enough to be empathetic, to listen to you, and to thoroughly evaluate and diagnose your problem. If your doctor or dentist downplays your problem or does not take it seriously, then you probably need to look for someone else who will and with whom you will feel more comfortable.

Your doctor or dentist needs to take time for a detailed medical history that will gather information about your physical and emotional health. These facts are very im-

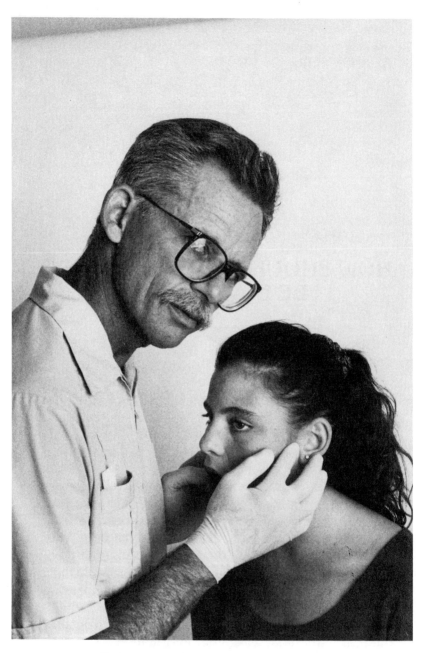

Palpating Joints For Pain And Noise

portant in placing your symptoms in a logical perspective. A good medical history should include information about your present symptoms, past illnesses, allergies, medical health, family medical problems, and various details regarding the social circumstances in your life, such as job interests, hobbies, alcohol and drug use, and causes of stress or anxiety in your life. Emotional and social factors are important because they can promote, aggravate, or alleviate pain. A good history will ask you about your chief complaints and when you first noticed them.

You should be asked to point to, or localize, where the pain or problem is coming from. You should be asked to describe the pain: whether it is sharp, dull, stabbing, burning, or throbbing. How long does the pain last? Does it last for seconds, minutes, or days? What makes the pain better? What makes it worse? Describe when you feel the pain during a typical 24-hour period. Rate the pain on a scale of 0 to 10, with 0 being no pain and 10 being the most pain that you could imagine.

Your doctor or dentist should then do a physical evaluation. He or she should evaluate your head and neck for any gross abnormalities: your posture, the way you hold your head over your shoulders, muscle tension, muscle development, and signs of stress or tension in your muscles. Your blood pressure should be recorded. Muscles of your head and neck should be palpated for signs of tenderness or soreness. Your temporomandibular joints should be palpated for signs of tenderness or soreness. Your joints should be listened to for evidence of noise, such as clicking, popping, or grating sounds. The movements of your joints should be recorded, such as how far you can open your mouth and how far you can move your jaw to the right, to the left, and forward. How much play there

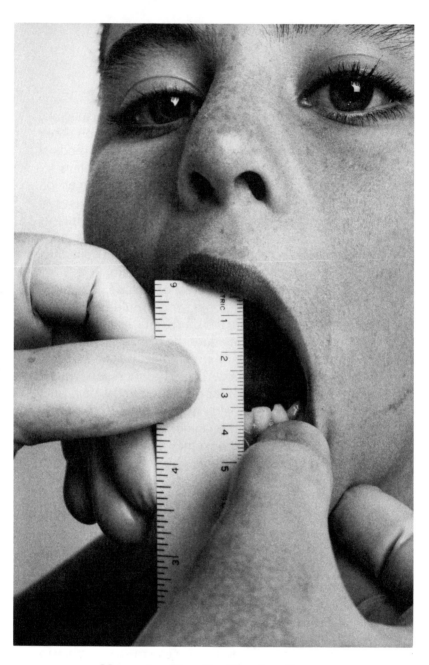

Measuring How Far The Jaw Opens

26

is in your joints, and what movements of your joints cause pain? Your mouth and teeth should be evaluated for signs of disease, and your teeth should be observed for signs of abnormal wear resulting from grinding your teeth.

Once all this information is compiled, your doctor or dentist will be able to come up with a clinical impression of what your problem is. He or she should explain the findings to you in such a way that you understand them and should take time to listen to your questions and give answers that are satisfactory to you.

Depending on how complicated your problem is, your doctor or dentist may need additional tests. The most common test is X-rays to evaluate the bones and joint for any abnormalities. Another test called a magnetic resonance imaging (MRI) study may be required to show the details of the soft tissues within the joint, such as the ligaments and the disc. Impressions of your teeth and jaws may be taken so that dental casts can be made to study the way your teeth are worn and meet. Your doctor or dentist may want to get consultations with other specialists, such as neurologists, to evaluate any nerve problems or possible tumors. Or a rheumatologist may be asked to evaluate the possibility of some type of arthritis. An ear, nose, and throat specialist could be asked to rule out problems of the ear. Even a psychologist could be consulted to evaluate your psychological status.

When all this information is gathered and evaluated, then your doctor or dentist will come up with a diagnosis. He or she will then talk to you about your diagnosis, about your prognosis, about the treatment, the alternatives to treatment, and specific recommendations. At this time you need to ask questions so that you thoroughly understand the proposed treatment, because for treatment to be successful, you must understand and participate in it.

TMJ Specialists

Most doctors and dentists can handle simple TMJ disorders. But if your TMJ problem is more complicated, or does not respond positively within a couple of weeks, you should seek the services of someone who is experienced in treating TMJ problems. Dentists are the health practitioners most experienced with TMJ problems, and there are dentists who specialize in treating TMJ disorders, even though this is not a recognized specialty. Most dental schools also have clinics specializing in TMJ problems. Often your family doctor or dentist will know of a dentist that is experienced in treating TMJ problems.

X-Rays and MRIs

Your dentist may want to take X-rays or use some other form of seeing the inside of your joint if it is likely that the problem is coming from your joint. If the problem is simply from your muscles, then you probably do not need X-rays.

There are two basic ways to see inside the joint. The first is through X-rays. X-rays are pictures taken using X-radiation. They are very good at showing hard tissues, that is, bone. Special X-rays called tomograms are used to look inside the joint and see the hard tissues. These X-rays will show structural abnormalities, fractures, and even tumors within the joint. They can also show abnormal wear of the joints, suggesting degenerative arthritis. But X-rays will show only the hard tissue or bones within the joint. They will not show the soft tissues, that is, the disc or ligaments

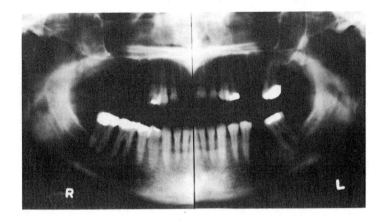

Panorex X-ray

within the joint. And TMJ problems are often due to injuries of the disc or ligaments.

In order to see the soft tissues within the joint, a process called magnetic resonance imaging (MRI) is used. This procedure uses no radiation. Your body is placed inside a tube that is surrounded by very powerful magnets. These magnets magnetize the water within your body, and then sound waves are passed through your body and give off pictures of the soft tissues inside the various structures of your body. This technique allows the soft tissues within the joint, namely, the disc and the ligaments, to be seen.

Both of these tests are quite expensive. TMJ X-rays cost about $200. An MRI costs about $800. Your dentist should order these tests only if they are necessary.

An additional disadvantage of X-rays is that they expose

one to a dose of harmful radiation. As we all know, we do not need any extra radiation and should have only radiation that can be justified in terms of possible benefits. Although an MRI study does not expose one to any harmful radiation, its main disadvantage is that you may need to keep your mouth open for up to 30 minutes, and this can aggravate an existing TMJ problem. Care needs to be taken during an MRI test to not open your mouth too wide and cause the muscles to go into spasm or to damage the joint ligaments. Another disadvantage is that some people are claustrophobic and can become afraid when enclosed in the MRI tube.

Other Tests

Electromyography

This is a technique that measures the electrical output of muscles in the face and neck by placing wires on the skin over the muscle to be tested. It is thought that excess electrical energy is an indication of stress and spasm. Scientifically it has not been proven to be a reliable test. Furthermore it gives you the same information you can obtain by palpating the muscle and seeing if the patient responds with pain.

Thermography

Thermography is a technique of measuring the skin temperature in an area of pain. Pain causes skin temperature changes. At the present it is being tested and has yet to be scientifically proven to be a reliable test. Therefore it is rarely used except in research.

Sonography

Sonography is the measuring and analyzing of the sounds made by a joint. At the present time this is still being tested. It could help to better our understanding of what causes sounds in the joint.

Doppler Auscultator

The Doppler is a stethoscope that magnifies the jaw joint sounds. One is able to hear much more detail about the sounds in the joint. It is usually not needed for diagnosis of TMJ problems. It can be useful for a surgeon if surgery is planned.

Jaw Recordings or Gnathogram

This is a graphic depiction of the movements of your jaw that can be used to document what is happening inside the joint. Such things as a displaced disc can be shown on these recordings. The same information can usually be shown by simple measurements of range of motion and clicking.

Notes

CHAPTER 4

HOW DOES THE TMJ WORK?

The temporomandibular joint is part of an interrelating system of bones, ligaments, muscles, nerves, teeth, and blood vessels. Each component of the system has an important job to do and each one relates to every other component. Like all systems, if one part is not functioning, then the system as a whole will function less than perfectly. In order to understand how the system functions, we need to look at each of the parts separately.

Bones

Two bones form the temporomandibular joint. One is the temporal bone, or skull bone. It has a concave socket, or fossa, into which fits the rounded end of the lower jawbone, called the mandible. Although these are the only bones in the joint itself, they are connected by muscles to many other bones. In the front of your neck, muscles connect the bottom of the jawbone to the hyoid bone,

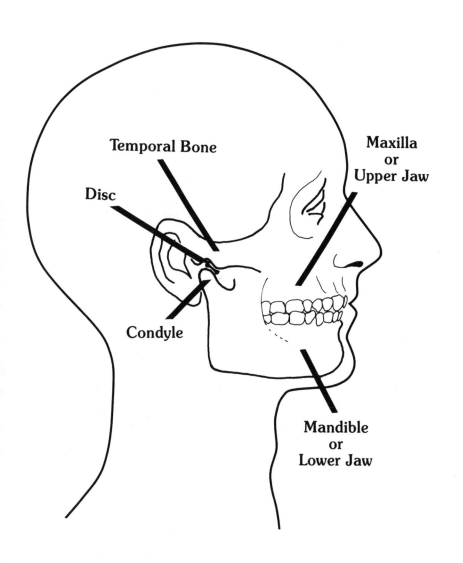

Temporal Bone

Maxilla
or
Upper Jaw

Disc

Condyle

Mandible
or
Lower Jaw

which you can feel in your neck when you swallow. Muscles from this bone connect to your collarbone. Muscles in the back of your neck attach to the back of your skull and down to the back of your neck and your shoulders.

Disc

Another important component of your temporomandibular joint is the disc, or pad, that fits between the two bones in the joint. This pad prevents the temporal bone and the mandible from rubbing on each other and wearing the bone away. The pad follows the bone in all movements and must slide wherever the bones slide. Any injury that displaces either disc so that it does not fit between the two bones can cause serious problems within the joint.

Ligaments

Ligaments hold the joint in place. These ligaments are called the capsule and tightly bind the joint so that it has stability. Other ligaments are also attached to the joint and surrounding bones to prevent the joint from over-opening and to give it more stability.

Synovial Fluid

The inside of the joint capsule is covered by a smooth membrane that produces a fluid that lubricates and protects the joint. It is necessary for that fluid to flow throughout the joint for proper lubrication. Movement of the joint helps to ciculate the synovial fluid, which enables

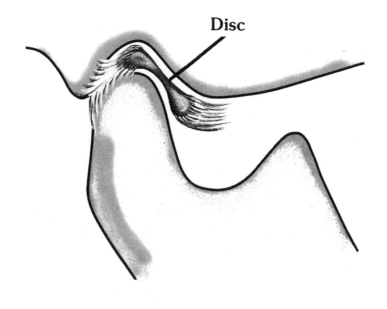

Disc

**Normal TMJ With Disc Acting As A
Cushion For Ball And Socket**

the joint to work smoothly. Injuries, stress, and arthritis can all affect the production and circulation of synovial fluid.

Muscles

There are many muscles in the TMJ system. First are the four chewing muscles. The first is the large cheek muscle (masseter), which you can feel when you clench your teeth together, right above your lower jaw. The next is the temple muscle (temporalis), which you can feel by placing your fingers on your temple when you clench your teeth together. Two other muscles on the inside of your jawbone help open and close your jaw and pull it forward. These are called the medial and lateral pterygoid muscles. These muscles need to be in balance and relaxed, except when they are at work.

The muscles in the front of your neck help you open your jaw. You can feel them by leaning your head far back and opening your jaw and feeling your neck. The muscles in the back of your neck are responsible for the position and posture of your head. If you lean your head forward, you can feel the tension in the muscles in the back of your neck. The muscles in the back of your neck need to be balanced with the muscles in the front of your neck so that your head is in the proper position and both sets of muscles are in a relaxed state.

Teeth

Another important component of this system are your teeth. They are attached to your lower jawbone and your upper jawbone and are controlled by the muscles, liga-

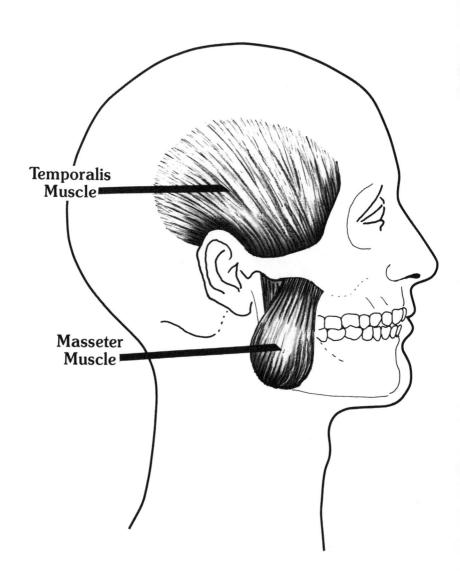

Temporalis Muscle

Masseter Muscle

Chewing Muscles On The Outside Of The Jaw

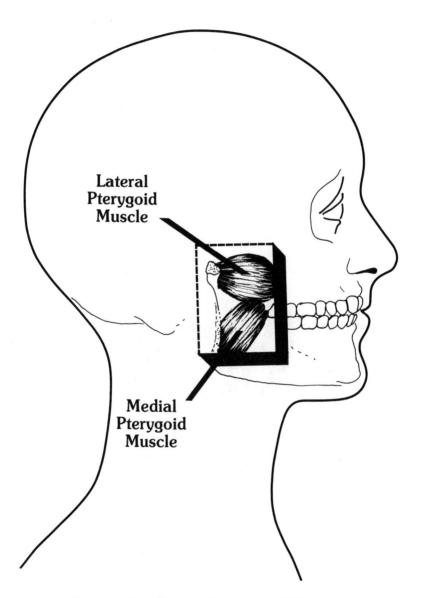

Lateral Pterygoid Muscle

Medial Pterygoid Muscle

Chewing Muscles On The Inside Of The Jaw

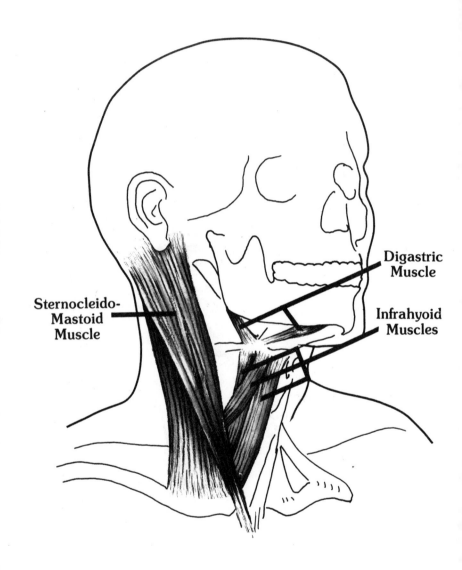

Digastric
Muscle

Sternocleido-
Mastoid
Muscle

Infrahyoid
Muscles

Muscles Of The Neck

40

ments, and discs. They fit together in a very precise manner.

Nerves

Nerves control the movements and feelings of the muscles, bones, teeth, and other parts of the system. Nerves coming from three of the neck vertebrae and three of the cranial nerves can refer pain to the TMJ. A complex network of nerves provides sensations to the neck, face, teeth, mouth, and tongue. It is no wonder that many patients complain of pain in their neck, ear, eyes, teeth, and head from TMJ disorders. Other sensory disturbances include dizziness, nausea, ringing in the ears, visual disturbances, loss of equilibrium, and numbness or tingling of face and hands.

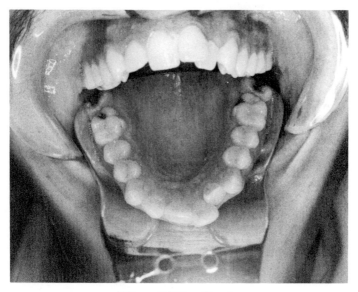

View Of Top Teeth

Blood Vessels

Blood vessels and lymph ducts help the health and vitality of all these parts. Blood vessels are also typically responsible for throbbing pains, a sign that something is wrong. When muscles contract and go into spasm, not enough blood goes to the muscles. This may cause throbbing pains in the muscle, joint, teeth or in other areas of the head and neck.

CHAPTER 5

WHAT CAUSES TMJ DISORDERS?

Most people think there are three major types of TMJ disorders: those involving the muscles, those involving the joint itself, and those involving the bite or the teeth. Most often there happens to be a combination of disorders.

Muscle Injuries

Many things cause injuries to the muscles, but probably number one is stress. Stress causes tension in muscles all over the body. Many backaches and neck aches, as most of us know, are caused by stress. And we can sometimes feel the muscles in our face tense up when we're under stress. Over time stress can cause the facial muscles to develop soreness and can also put pressure on the TMJ and make the joint sore.

Clenching and grinding of the teeth, or bruxism, is another cause of sore muscles. This clenching and grind-

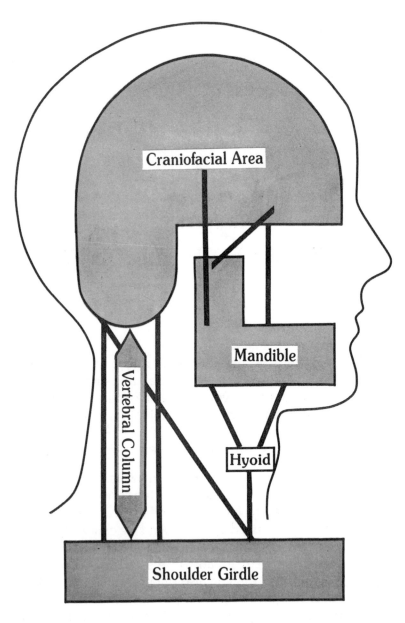

Diagram Showing Balance Of Head On Vertebral Column
And How Muscles Stabilize The System

44

ing can put abnormal stresses on the muscles, which causes them to become sore. Bruxism can also cause the joint to become sore. Bruxism is microtrauma.

Trauma, or injuries to the muscles, can also cause soreness. Often people who are hit in the face or jaw by a fist, in a fall, or in an automobile accident get sore facial muscles. When the muscles are stretched beyond their normal length, they can be damaged, bruised, or torn.

Joint Injuries

The main cause of damage to the joint is probably trauma or injuries. The jaw joint can be torn and damaged just like a knee or ankle joint. Ligaments can be torn, discs can be displaced, and the joint itself can be bruised and injured in other ways.

Earaches and headaches can also be caused by problems coming from the temporomandibular joint. When the joint is injured through trauma such as a blow to the jaw, or through traumatic overuse, such as excessive grinding of teeth at night it can become painful. Inflammation and swelling take place within the joint and this causes pain.

Damage to the internal structures of the joint, such as the disc or ligaments, can also cause pain.

Danger on the Freeway

Charlotte had been in a severe automobile accident. Someone had stopped in front of her on the freeway, and she had to come to a quick stop to avoid hitting him. But the car behind her did not see her stopping and plowed into her car, going about 30 miles per hour. Her head was thrown back violently and then went forward and hit the dashboard. She had no cuts and only a bruise on her forehead where she hit the dashboard. She was taken to the hospital to be checked out and was found to have pain in her back, neck, and jaw.

She came to see me three days later. Her complaints were pain in her jaw, head, and neck and an inability to open her mouth without a click in her jaw. I found both her temporomandibular joints very sore, and the muscles in her face, cheek, and temple area as well as the back of her neck were very sore to touch. And she could only open her mouth about one and a half fingers' width. To open it wider, she had to jiggle her jaw to make it pop. In addition to injuring the joint and muscles, Charlotte had had the disc, or pad, that fits between her lower jaw and the base of her skull displaced forward or anteriorly. (This type of injury is called an anterior displaced disc, or an internal derangement.) It can be more serious than other types of temporomandibular joint injuries because the disc is no longer in the location that it should be for proper functioning of the jaw. The body then has to go through a healing process of forming scar tissue out of the injured tissue so that the jaw can function on scar tissue and be able to use that as a disc. This injury can take up to several years to heal. In some cases it can be a chronic problem and never be quite right.

Charlotte was treated with a soft diet, physical therapy, anti-inflamatory medication, and a splint. After about six months, her symptoms were almost gone. She continues to wear her splint at night, and when her symptoms start to reappear, she goes back to eating soft foods and applying heat and ice to her joint. As as result, she has managed to be largely pain free.

Whiplash

Whiplash injuries in automobile accidents are a common cause of injury to the joint. In a whiplash injury, the head is thrown back and the lower jaw is pulled forward, causing a tearing of the ligaments in the joint. Whiplash injuries also can injure the muscles and ligaments of the neck and shoulders.

Bad Bites

Problems with your bite are less apt to cause problems with your TMJ than is stress or injury. Studies have shown that people with abnormal bites do not have any higher incidence of TMJ problems than people with normal bites.

Watch for High Bridges

Mary had had some of her back teeth extracted years earlier. She went to a dentist who suggested that she have her missing teeth replaced with bridges. After she had bridges made, Mary noticed that she started getting headaches and earaches and was very concerned. Her dentist gave her medication, which helped only for a short while. She went back to her dentist, complaining of the headaches, and he referred her to a neurologist. The neurologist gave her medication for the headaches, which helped somewhat but she felt

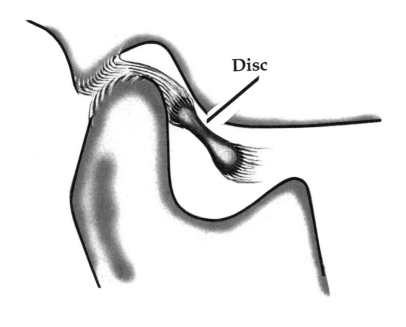

Disc

**TMJ With Disc Displaced Forward, Or Anteriorly,
With The Loss Of The Cushion Between The Two Bones**

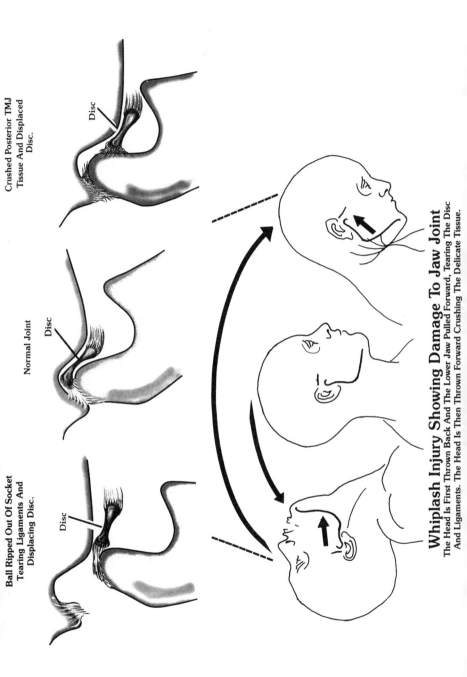

Crushed Posterior TMJ Tissue And Displaced Disc.

Disc

Normal Joint

Disc

Ball Ripped Out Of Socket Tearing Ligaments And Displacing Disc.

Disc

Whiplash Injury Showing Damage To Jaw Joint
The Head Is First Thrown Back And The Lower Jaw Pulled Forward, Tearing The Disc And Ligaments. The Head Is Then Thrown Forward Crushing The Delicate Tissue.

49

so drowsy that it was very difficult for her to carry out the functions of her job and live a normal life. She suffered with these headaches for over a year and finally went to another dentist. He found her headaches were, in fact, coming from her right temporomandibular joint, which was very sore to touch, as were the muscles in the cheek and temple area. Her bridge was too high, which caused her bite to be off. The bridge was removed, and her symptoms immediately improved. This is an example of a bite that was suddenly changed.

One of the major causes of TMJ problems resulting from bad bites is dental work. Many people who have had their jaws repositioned or have had extensive crown and bridge work to change their bites have ended up having problems with their TMJ. Surgery to the jaw, or even a broken jaw, may dramatically change the way your teeth meet, which can lead to TMJ problems.

However, most people with bad bites have had them for their entire lives and have adjusted to them. Even though your bite may need to be fixed so that you can chew better and have a more stable bite, more and more studies are showing that your bite is probably not the cause of most TMJ problems.

The goal for a patient with a TMJ disorder and a bad bite is to enable the patient to be pain free and be able to function with his/her jaws. Some patients will need to learn how to manage their TMJ problem so that they can live a normal life. The treatment should accomplish these goals without changing their bad bite in an irreversible way. Only after a patient has been comfortable for some period of time — at least six months — should any correction of the "bad bite" be attempted. It is important to remember that the bad bite is being corrected for dental reasons, that is, a healthier and more functional mouth. It is not for treating the TMJ disorder. This has already been accomplished. The patient is relatively pain free and can use his or her jaw in a normal way. The patient will need to manage his/her problem for the rest of their lives regardless of whether or not their bite is corrected for dental reasons.

Sudden Bite Changes

Loss of the back or molar teeth can cause the jaw to collapse. The molar teeth provide support against the strong forces of the chewing muscles. If the back teeth are lost and not replaced the forces of the muscles can cause the jaw to be pulled higher up into the socket. This can place a strain on the tissues inside the joint. It is good dental practice to have extracted teeth replaced in order to prevent this collapse.

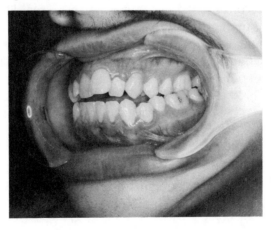

Bad Bite — Front Teeth Do Not Meet

Arthritis and Other Diseases

Many degenerative diseases that affect other joints in the body, such as arthritis, can often affect the TMJ. Developmental problems with the TMJ causing one joint to grow larger than the other can also cause problems. Tumors, both benign and malignant, can affect the TMJ, but these are rare. Many disorders of other parts of the body can refer pain to the face and TMJ. Neck injuries or neck muscle pain can be felt in the TMJ and can affect the muscles of the TMJ. Problems with nerves can be felt as pain in the TMJ or the face. Pain from your heart can also be referred to your jaw area. Certain drugs and medication can also have an effect on your TMJ and muscles. Psychological disorders can also affect your TMJ, and especially affect the way that pain affects you.

As you can see, there can be many causes of TMJ and facial pain problems. You need to see a doctor or a dentist to have your pain diagnosed and to rule out the possibility of any serious causes. Also, in real life, most problems are combinations of several causes. Therefore, it may take time and a lot of investigation to finally find out what causes your specific problems and how to treat them most effectively.

Stress and Distress

The Headaches Made Me Cry

Susan had a lot of stress in her life. She had seen her doctor for headaches and earaches that were so severe at times they made her cry. She was referred for a CAT scan to rule out any kind of tumor that might have been causing these severe headaches. She had seen a chiropractor but had not gotten any relief from that treatment. She came to me because she thought that a tooth might be causing these bad headaches. Susan had very sore joints, and her muscles in her temple and cheek area were very sore. She had worn her teeth flat from grinding them at night. She stated that she would wake up in the morning with her jaws tight and sore and feeling like they were locked together, and she would usually have a headache.

Susan's headaches were due to overworking her muscles and TMJ by grinding her teeth at night. I recommended a soft diet, aspirin for the pain and inflammation in her joints and muscles, and the use of heat and ice, and I urged her to try to reduce the stress in her life. In addition, she began to use a splint to prevent her from placing the tremendous forces on her joints and muscles when she ground her teeth. The splint also acted as a reminder that she was clenching her teeth. After following the treatment and wearing her splint for about a month, her pain disappeared. She has remained pain free over the past year and manages her problem. When her TMJ starts to act up, she then returns to a soft diet, heat, ice, aspirin, and recognizing the stress in her life to head off the severe headaches that bothered her before.

Stress plays a very significant role in TMJ problems. What is stress? Stress can be either physical or emotional. The body cannot tell the difference. Stress is usually due to the fight-or-flight syndrome. All animals, including humans, have this response. The automatic nervous system triggers

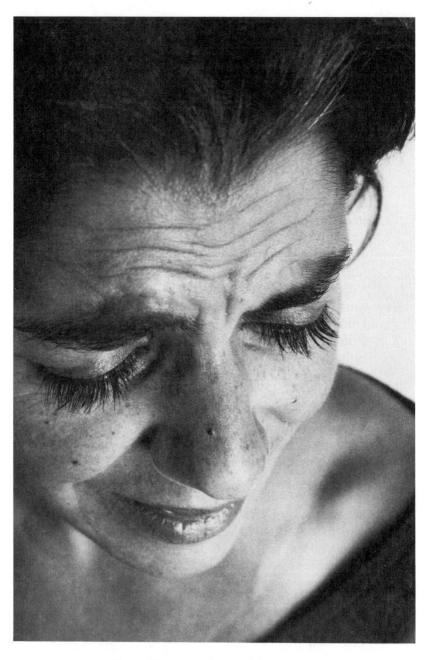

Face Showing Signs Of Distress

this complicated neurological and chemical reaction of the body to danger. Chemicals, like adrenalin, are released to make us able to run faster. Blood vessels are constricted on the outer surfaces of the body, making more blood go to the internal organs and the heart so that the body can perform faster, enabling a protective response.

An antelope fleeing for its life from a lion is an example of a classical fight-or-flight syndrome response. People often respond with superhuman efforts in times of extreme danger. This too is an example of the fight-or-flight response. Almost everyone, especially athletes, has responded under stress or pressure at some time and has used this automatic-nervous-system response to perform at a higher level than normal.

As you can see by these examples, it is necessary and good that we can respond in stressful situations. Stress becomes harmful when it becomes chronic or long-term. Then it is called distress. Nature intended the stress response to be used only occasionally and only for a short time, as, for example, in fleeing from a life-threatening situation. When stress is prolonged, it becomes negative and harmful. Examples of harmful, prolonged stress or distress can be seen in animals that are in captivity in zoos. Because of the distress, many of these animals die or undergo other changes, such as not being able to breed in captivity.

Most distress in modern-day society is emotional stress: the death of a loved one, the loss of a job, a big test, an important social function, or being caught in traffic on your way to an important appointment. Even positive events, like marriage or pregnancy, can be stressful. Life is full of many stressful situations, and it is important that we be able

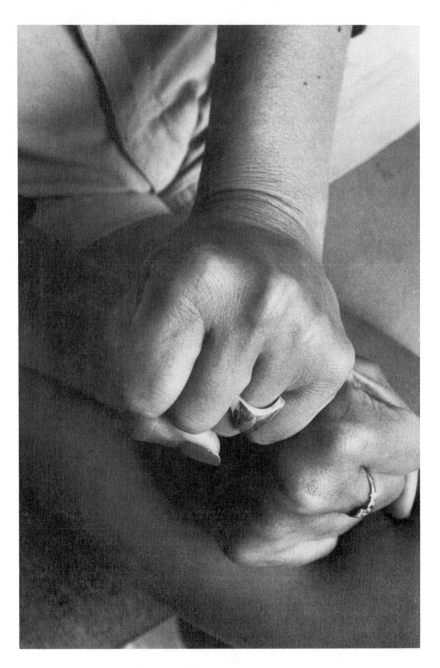

Hands Showing Distress

to deal with them. You can measure the distress in your life, using the Life Stress Scale shown at the end of this chapter.

We all know some of the harmful effects that stress can have on our health, such as stomach ulcers, high blood pressure, skin rashes, and various emotional disorders. Studies have shown that stress over a long period of time can also reduce the response of the immune system. Most of us know either personally or from other people how much more susceptible one is to various illness when one is under long-term stress.

So, how does distress affect the temporomandibular joint? Imagine what a person under chronic stress would look like. First, the jaw muscles would be clenched together tightly, with the teeth touching each other. The facial muscles would be tightened and the brow might be furrowed. The muscles around the eyes and face would be scrunched up together. The neck and shoulder muscles would be very tight.

Take a few seconds and put yourself in this stress posture. Clench your teeth and tighten your shoulder, neck and facial muscles. You may even feel the rest of your body joining in. Your fists may clench and your legs may tighten up. This is an example of a stress response, and if it is continued over a long period of time, it can have harmful effects on your TMJ.

Prolonged clenching of your jaw muscles can cause the structures inside the joint to be damaged and either to swell up or to become inflamed. The disc that fits between the lower jawbone and the skull can even be squeezed and pushed out of shape from prolonged clenching or muscle tension. Clenching and grinding your teeth can also have harmful effects on the internal structures of your jaw.

Muscles that are tensed for long periods of time can become sore, can get knots in them, and can even go into spasm. It is easy to see how stress can have a deleterious effect on your TMJ.

Sometimes stress may not affect your TMJ immediately and noticeably, but it can make it a weak spot. For example, if you have a car accident and injure your TMJ, then the injury added to the effects of earlier stress may trigger a serious TMJ problem.

In short, stress is intimately related to all TMJ problems and must be controlled in order to get rid of TMJ pain.

Life Stress Scale

Major changes in your life cause stress and can make you more susceptible to illness, including TMJ pain. This scale can help you recognize when you are under unusual stress. In the stressful periods of your life, you need to take especially good care of yourself.

To determine your life stress score, add up the number of stress units for each event that you have experienced during the last year. A score of 150 points for events occurring within the last year means a 50 percent chance of developing an illness. A score of 300 means a 90 percent chance.

Event Stress Units Score

Event	Score
Death of a spouse	100
Divorce	73
Marital separation	63
Jail term	63
Death of close family member	63

What Causes TMJ Disorders?

Personal injury or illness 53
Marriage 50
Fired from work 47
Marital reconciliation 45
Retirement 45
Change in health of family member 44
Pregnancy 40
Sex difficulties 39
Gain of new family member 39
Business readjustment 39
Change in financial state 38
Death of close friend 37
Change to different line of work 36
Change in number of arguments w/spouse . . 35
Mortgage over $10,000* 31
Foreclosure of mortgage or loan 30
Change in responsibilities at work 29
Son or daughter leaving home 29
Trouble with in-laws 29
Outstanding personal achievement 28
Spouse begins or stops work 26
Begin or end school 26
Change in living conditions 25
Revision of personal habits 24
Trouble with boss 23
Change in work hours or conditions 20
Change in residence 20
Change in schools 20
Change in recreation 19
Change in church activities 19
Change in social activities 18
Mortgage or loan less than $10,000* 17
Change in sleeping habits 16

Change in number of family get-togethers . . .   15
Change in eating habits   15
Vacation   13
Christmas   12
Minor violations of the law   11

TOTAL _____

* Because this scale was developed in 1967, the amount of mortgage cost should be adjusted to current prices, probably about $100,000 in most parts of the country.

Source: Holmes and Rahe, "The Social Readjustment Rating Scale." *Journal of Psychosomatic Research* 2 (1967): 213-218.

Bruxism

A Case of Grinding Your Teeth

Dorothy, who was in her mid 50s, had been having daily headaches for the past ten years. It seemed she would wake up every morning with a headache. She had discussed this with many doctors over the years and had been given various types of pain medication but none seemed to help very much. When I examined her, both of her temporomandibular joints were very sore to touch as were the chewing muscles in her cheeks and temple area. From her history we concluded that Dorothy was grinding her teeth at night due to stress. This caused her muscles and joints to become sore and she would wake up with a headache. We discussed various forms of treatment, including wearing a splint at night so that she would not place destructive forces on her muscles and joint, but she did not want to wear one. We decided to try an antidepressant medication called Elavil (or Amitriptyline). It works by altering sleep patterns and causing a deeper stage of sleep so that people do not grind their teeth during sleep. It also affects the central nervous system and seems to reduce pain.

Dorothy was given very small doses of Elavil — 10 milligrams — and was to take one tablet at bedtime each night. I saw her two weeks after she began taking the tablets, and her headaches had completely disappeared. We cut her dose back to one tablet only on those nights when she felt she was under somewhat more stress than usual. At the end of several weeks she had had two or three headaches, but they had been much less severe. She felt that this was something that she could live with — that is, having one not-too-severe headache every week or ten days.

Bruxism is the grinding and clenching of the teeth during sleep. Many people are not aware that they grind or clench their teeth; the only evidence is that they wake up with a sore jaw or the person who sleeps next to them complains about the noise they make from grinding their teeth.

Studies have shown that clenching your jaw muscle for ninety seconds will fatigue the muscle and cause pain. A typical pattern of grinding at night is to clench your teeth five times for one second and then continually clench for about twenty seconds. This will be repeated several times throughout the night. Probably 95 percent of us clench and grind our teeth at some time during our life. If this totals no more than two or three minutes per night, as in most cases, probably there will be little if any discomfort. But some people continuously contract their jaw muscles for up to three minutes at a time, and during the night they may exceed forty minutes of contracting their muscles. This type of overuse, especially if the jaw is in an awkward position, can cause severe muscle and joint pain.

People who brux do not do it the same amount every night. Long-term studies have shown that they will grind their teeth in a more normal pattern for two or three weeks and then over a period of one to many days will go into a pattern of excessive grinding and clenching. These episodes of abnormal grinding seem to be related to times of stress. When the stress eases, they will then resume a more normal pattern of grinding their teeth at night.

Many dentists used to think that people ground their teeth because their teeth did not meet right. Teeth are supposed to function smoothly, like gears, without interferences. Because dentists thought that interferences caused people to grind their teeth, they often treated bruxism by grinding the interferences off the teeth. But studies of people sleeping with interferences put on their teeth have shown that, in fact, the opposite is true. People grind and clench their teeth less when interferences are placed on their teeth.

This finding led to further study of bruxism to discover why people grind and clench their teeth. Electrodes were placed on people's facial muscles while they slept to find out how much grinding was done, and why. What was shown is that people grind more during periods of stress. The conclusion of the scientific studies is that stress is the primary cause of night grinding and clenching of teeth. These same studies have also shown that certain medications that reduce stress, such as tranquilizers and antidepressant medications, can reduce the amount of grinding.

Other drugs, however, can also increase bruxism. For

example, people who abuse amphetamines tend to grind and clench their teeth more. Heavy use of alcohol also increases grinding.

Treatments

Are there any ways of stopping bruxism during the night? Dentists used to think that placing a plastic splint between the teeth during the night would stop bruxism. But studies in which electrodes were placed on people's muscles during sleep while they were wearing splints have shown that this is not true. People grind their teeth just as much with splints as they do without them. What splints do is minimize the amount of pressure placed on the joints. They will not stop bruxism, but they can protect the joints and teeth from the harmful effects of grinding during the night.

Studies have been done with nocturnal biofeedback. This is a method where wires on your facial muscles are connected to a beeper, and when you grind your teeth, the beeper starts beeping. The studies have shown that people stop grinding as soon as the beeper sounds. But this biofeedback method works only while the person is wearing the beeper. When there is nothing to alert the person to tooth grinding, it resumes as before.

Bruxism in Children

Bruxism isn't a problem only of adults under stress. Children grind their teeth too — sometimes very loudly. My clinical observations indicate that almost all children grind their baby teeth so that they are relatively flattened. But very few children have pain in their facial muscles or joints from this type of grinding. Bruxism is so common

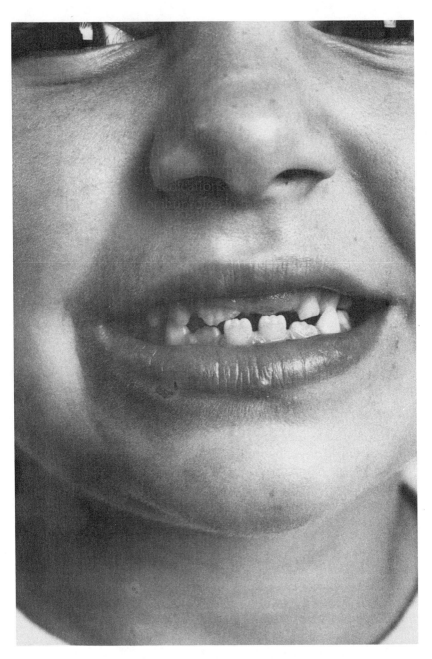

Children Often Grind Their Teeth

among children that it is unlikely to be related to stress. It seems to be related to the permanent teeth growing underneath the baby teeth and pushing them out. The permanent teeth are putting pressure on the baby teeth, and the roots of the baby teeth are dissolving. Children often complain of pressure in their baby teeth and sometimes of mild pain from the eruptive forces of the permanent teeth. It is my opinion that grinding of baby teeth is some part of a natural process to help push them out so that they can be replaced by the permanent teeth.

Sex

Not Tonight, I have An Aching Jaw

Marlene had had a chronic problem with her TMJ for years and had managed it well, but the problem would get worse from time to time. She was able to take care of these episodes herself by using some of the techniques that she had learned, such as using heat, ice, and rest. I had not seen her for quite some time when she came in again complaining of pain in her jaw. The examination revealed that she had mostly soreness of her joint and a decrease in the opening of her jaw. She related to me that she had just returned from her honeymoon and felt that being very sexually active and engaging in oral sex had strained her jaw. We discussed this, and after she had abstained from oral sex for three weeks, her jaw and pain became much better and she became asymptomatic.

Oral sex can be bad for your TMJ. During oral sex people often keep their mouth in an uncomfortable position for long periods of time, either opening it abnormally wide or placing it in a position that the muscles are not used to. This can cause both the muscles and the joint to become sore or to aggravate an already sore muscle or joint problem.

Kissing can also aggravate TMJ problems. Especially passionate kissing over a long period of time can place abnormal forces on the joint and utilize muscles that are not normally used. This can make both the joint and muscles sore.

Should you avoid kissing and oral sex? No. You have to be practical about this. Sex can be great for reducing stress, and we have seen that stress is one of the major contributors to TMJ problems. If your TMJ is very sore, and you are trying to let it heal, then you probably should avoid anything, including oral sex and passionate kissing, that tends to make it worse. When your TMJ gets better, then you can gradually return to these types of sexual activity. But gradualness is the key, because overexertion of any muscle after a period of inactivity can aggravate a healing injury or cause the muscles to become sore.

CHAPTER 6

WHAT CAUSES TMJ SYMPTOMS?

Pain and noises in the joints of the jaw are common symptoms. Pain can be caused by swelling or inflammation of the joint, pressure on the tissues when the disc has been displaced, or arthritis of the joint.

But it is important to note that joint noises alone do not necessarily mean that your jaw or joint needs to be treated. Sounds only give an indication as to what the problem is. Unless the sound is associated with either pain or inability to function, such as being unable to open or close your mouth, it is not usually a reason for treatment.

Joint Noises and Joint Pain

Structural Abnormality

Your jaw can pop or click for several reasons. Probably the most common one is a structural abnormality in the joint itself. The joint will rise up over the abnormal struc-

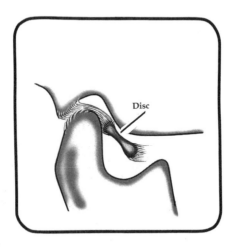

Jaw Closed With Disc Displaced Forward

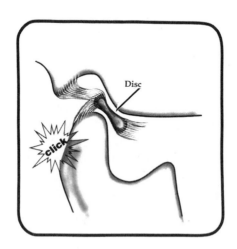

**Clicking Sound Is Made When Jaw Opens
And Pops Up Onto Displaced Disc**

ural defect every time the jaw is opened and closed. This causes a noise, either a popping or clicking sound. It does not mean that there is anything wrong with the jaw other than the structural abnormality that causes it to pop or click.

Over-Opening

Another reason that the jaw can pop is if it is opened too wide; the jaw can go out over the socket and cause a popping sound. In this case, the jaw pops only at the most wide-open position and also pops at the same place when you attempt to close it. This kind of popping does not necessarily indicate that anything is wrong, but repeated over-opening can stretch the ligaments in the joint and cause your jaw to lock open and not be able to be closed. It is not good to overstretch the ligaments in a joint.

Displaced Disc

A displaced disc is another reason that a jaw pops or clicks. If the disc is pulled forward as you open, your jaw will pop or click up onto the disc and then as you close, it may pop or click back off of the disc. This is because the disc has been pulled or torn and is in a forward position. A displaced disc is often caused by trauma, such as a car accident or a blow to the jaw.

Sticking Disc

Another cause of a clicking or popping sound is a sticking disc. This can be caused by nighttime clenching or grinding your teeth that squashes the disc flat and presses all the lubrication out of it. Upon awakening, the disc will not move smoothly and the jawbone may slide off of the disc.

As the jaw is moved about, lubrication can again flow around the disc. The disc then is able to move with the jaw, and the popping or clicking sound will disappear.

Headaches

Headaches, like backaches, are most likely caused by muscle tension and muscle spasm. When your jaw muscles become sore they can cause headaches. Also, muscles in the head and neck that go into spasm or have sore knots in them can refer pain to areas of the head and face away from the muscle itself. Neck aches can be caused by muscles in the neck that are sore. When your jaw muscles are going into spasm, they often influence the neck muscles to become sore, too. Poor posture will cause the facial and neck muscles to be out of balance and contract and become sore and then ache. This will often give rise to neck aches and headaches.

Earaches

Earaches are another matter. The TMJ is just in front of the ear. Pain inside the joint of the TMJ can be referred to the ear. Many of the same nerves that go to the joint also go to the ear. Patients often complain of earache when, in fact, the ache is in their TMJ.

Muscle Aches

Why do muscles hurt? Most of you have experienced muscle cramps and can understand why a contracted muscle hurts. In addition, other parts of the muscles, such as the blood vessels and tendons, can become inflamed and cause the muscle to ache. In muscle pain, there is

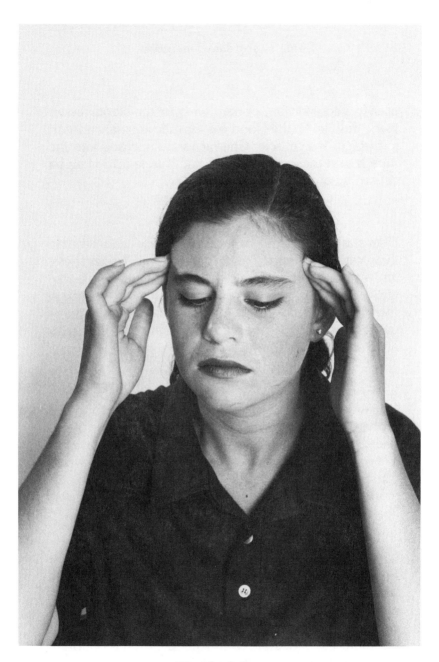

Muscle Aches

usually a constriction, or narrowing, of the blood vessels in the muscle. Or the blood vessels may enlarge and start to throb in the muscle. Chemicals are released into the muscle and these also cause pain. Muscle aches can be caused by a number of factors.

Distress

Distress is one of the major causes of muscle aches because it can cause muscles to contract and tighten. Under stress, turtles retract their neck and head into their shell as a protective response. Humans do a similar thing by retracting their head and neck into their shoulders when they're under stress. This response to stress tightens the muscles and causes them to undergo spasm.

Pain

Pain is another cause of tension or muscle ache. You can probably relate to having had pain somewhere in your body and feeling your muscles tense up. This can give rise to a cycle of muscle spasm, which causes more pain, which causes more muscle spasm. This cycle can become so profound that it perpetuates itself, even after the original cause has been stopped.

Poor Posture

Posture can also affect muscles. We have probably all felt muscle ache when a part of our body has been in an uncomfortable position for a long period of time. Some people respond as they do to stress by retracting the head back into the shoulders. Other people do the opposite. They hold their neck and head forward in a strained posi-

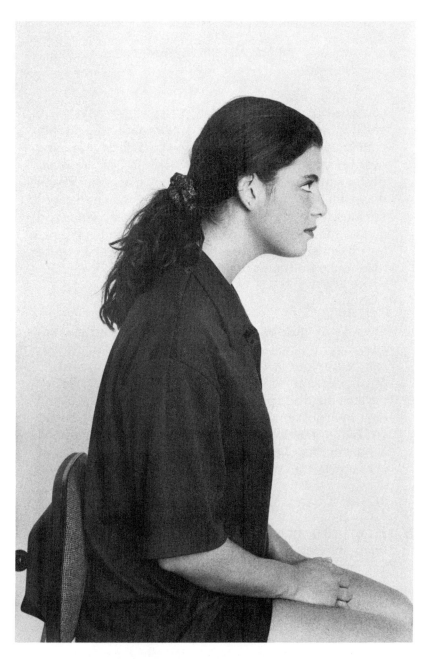

Poor Sitting Posture — Head Forward

tion when in a tense situation such as driving a car in heavy traffic or bad weather. Sitting in an awkward position with your head forward and your jaw on your chest or leaning over on your side to watch TV while in bed are other postural positions that can cause muscle aches. Looking down while reading or working at a desk can also cause the muscles in the back of the neck to become tense and go into spasm. Stretching your neck backward and looking up working under a car or painting ceilings can cause pain in the front part of your neck muscles.

Overuse

Overuse of muscles can also cause them to ache. Gum chewing or prolonged chewing of very hard or tough foods can cause your jaw muscles to ache and become sore. Many people at night overwork their jaw muscles by grinding their teeth and placing their jaws in uncomfortable and abnormal positions while they are asleep. This prolonged use of the muscles can cause them to become sore and ache. You may wake up in the morning finding that your jaw muscles are sore.

What Is Pain?

Pain, like beauty, is in the eye of the beholder. What is painful to one person may not be painful to another or may be experienced in a different way. Pain is something that only the person who is experiencing it understands.

Pain is very much like stress. It is controlled by part of the automatic nervous system. When your hand touches a hot stove, your brain instantly feels pain and the hand jerks back. This is an automatic response to protect you from serious injury. If you did not feel the pain, your hand might become badly burned. Acute pain causes a fight-or-flight reaction in the human body.

Pain is a message that something is wrong. It can cause anxiety, which is a natural response to pain. Pain is telling the body not to use that part in order to allow it to heal. When a person feels pain and cannot find the cause, the result is anxiety. Once the cause of the pain is discovered, usually the anxiety is reduced and then the pain is reduced. There is a relationship between anxiety and pain. The higher the anxiety, the more the pain is felt.

When pain becomes chronic, it becomes similar to stress. Like chronic stress, chronic pain can become damaging both physically and psychologically. Animals that experience chronic pain crawl away and lay down and die. That is nature's way of dealing with mortal illness and injuries. In humans, the same sort of response takes place. People with chronic pain — that is, pain that lasts over six months — show sleep disturbances, loss of appetite, irritability, withdrawal of social interests, and other signs of depression. Psychological testing of chronic-pain patients usually shows them to be depressed, and it has also been shown that treatment of depression often results in a reduction in the amount of pain perceived. The pain causes more stress, then the stress causes more pain, and then the more pain causes further stress. This cycle repeats itself and becomes essentially a self-perpetuating mechanism. Thus, treating stress and depression is absolutely necessary in treating pain.

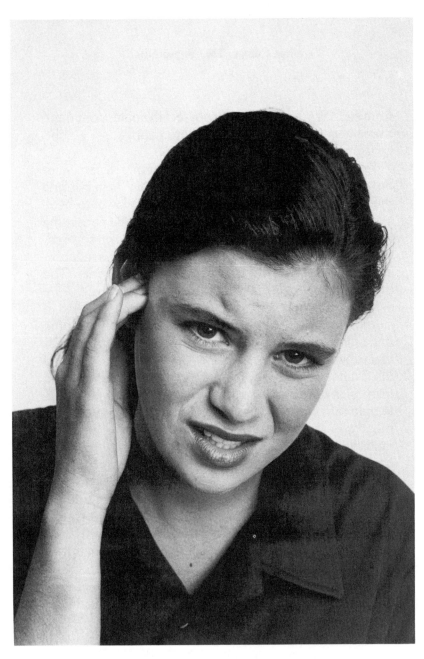

Pain In Temporomandibular Joint (TMJ)

EMOTIONAL AND PSYCHOLOGICAL EFFECTS OF TMJ PAIN

Pain is subjective. Only you know exactly how pain feels to you. Pain is influenced by your emotions. Your mind exerts a very strong influence on how you respond to pain. For example, an injury occurring while doing something enjoyable may not hurt very much at the time and you may not notice it until later, when the pain becomes apparent. The opposite is also very common. You may notice an injury just before you are about to do something unpleasant and the pain may, in fact, be out of proportion to the injury. It may be an unconscious excuse to avoid the unpleasant activity.

Your pain threshold is influenced by your emotional state. Pain threshold has been described as a biological thermostat that regulates where you feel pain at any given time. Depression, anxiety, and frustration all decrease the pain threshold, or make it so that less pain is felt sooner. In contrast, happiness, enjoyment, and feelings of well being all raise the pain threshold.

Your present feelings about pain are influenced by whether you got attention and love in your childhood for pain and illness. Many children got extra attention and needed love whenever they were sick and thus learned that sickness and illness brought about love and attention. Children often experience a minor illness, such as stomach ache or headache, when they have to do things that they do not want to, such as go to school. They learn from an early age that illness or pain can be used to avoid unpleasant things.

Even into adulthood, many people use illness and pain as an escape from the burdens of life. For example, an

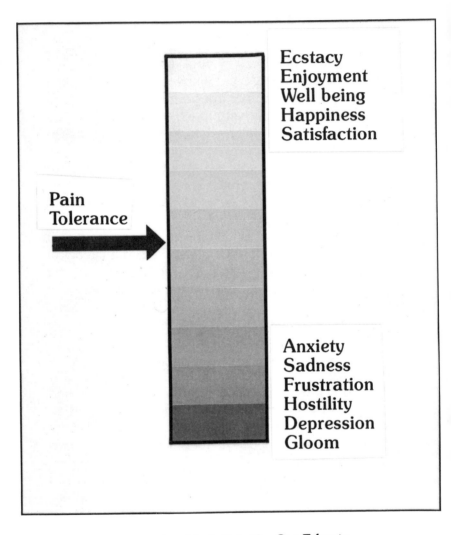

Pain Scale. How Much Pain You Can Tolerate
Is Relative To How Good You Feel

overworked mother may get relief from the stress of caring for children and household chores only by illness or pain. Or pain or illness may be the only relief from the rigors of a job or school. Pain or sickness can result in sympathy, rest, medication, and time off work.

Psychological factors can also influence illness or pain when a person has an injury that is being litigated. The amount of the settlement is in part determined by how serious the injury is, how much pain it causes, and how much disability there is. Therefore, it is in the interest of the injured person not to heal and not to get well. Very few patients I have seen do this on a conscious level, but unconsciously, it plays a significant role. When we focus on an injury, we tend to increase our awareness of it. I have seen many patients not make much improvement until a settlement has been reached and they are able to let go of the injury and get on with their life.

Pain and illness allow some people the gratification of dependency on a parent figure, such as their doctor or their spouse. Continuation of the pain and illness gives them the gratification of that relationship. Patients need to take responsibility for their own recovery and utilize the help of others to get well, not to stay sick.

Pain of the unknown can be exaggerated. Fear increases pain as many people think of the worst. When the cause of pain is diagnosed and explained, the pain diminishes or even disappears. The pain has served its natural purpose of warning you that something is wrong.

Cultural factors are closely related to emotional factors. These factors from one's background can also have an influence on the way people interpret pain. Different cultures interpret pain and illness in different ways, as do men and women.

There is a lot we do not know about how pain and illness are influenced by emotional and psychological factors. But we do know that the relationship exists. How these influences are brought to bear depends upon each individual.

CHAPTER 7

SELF-CARE TIPS FOR TMJ DISORDERS

I Can't Chew Hard Foods

Burt came to me complaining of pain whenever he ate hard foods. The pain would radiate up to his ear and to the temple area of his head and make it impossible for him to chew anything harder than scrambled eggs. When I examined him, I found both of his temporomandibular joints were sore to touch and his muscles in the temple and cheek area were also very sore. Burt was instructed to adhere to a soft diet in order to rest his sore joints and muscles and allow them to heal. After two weeks of eating nothing but a soft diet, he was able to gradually increase the hardness of the food that he ate until he was back to a normal diet. He learned to manage his jaw problem by managing the type and hardness of the food that he ate. From time to time when his jaw would act up, he would then have to resort to eating a softer diet, cutting his food in smaller pieces and chewing it on his back teeth for a day or two until his jaw felt better and he could start easing into a more normal diet. He has been able to manage his jaw pain for several years this way.

Once you have a diagnosis and an explanation of the problem, your understanding will help you deal with this problem. You will understand that you have a weakness or disability in your TMJ, and this most likely will be with you for the rest of your life. When you learn how to take care of it, you will be able to live with it. But if you do not take care of it, if you do things that are harmful to your TMJ, especially during periods of stress, you will then have problems with it.

Throughout the rest of your life, you will have to pay close attention to your body. When it gives you the message that there is pain in some part of it, it is telling you not to use that part. It is telling you to rest it, to take care of it, to let it heal.

Living with TMJ problems is similar to living with back problems because you can manage both of them. People with back problems need to know how to lift and how to move, how to have good posture, how to prevent their back from flaring up. If their back does start to flare up, they then need to take action to prevent it from getting worse. This is how people with back problems manage their problems. Much work has been done with backs in the past decade, and people now rarely have to undergo the surgery that was quite common years ago.

1. Rest

If you have pain, your body is telling you to not use your TMJ. You need to let it heal. The way you do that is to rest it. Rest means to give it minimal use and to do nothing that will make the condition worse. The normal resting position for your TMJ and facial muscles is with the teeth apart and the lips relaxed, either just parted or lightly together.

2. Soft Diet

When trying to allow an injured TMJ to heal, you need to adhere to a soft diet. Hard foods put a tremendous strain on your jaw joint and muscles and can delay healing or cause a worsening of the situation. Especially to be avoided are hard foods, chewy tough meats, and tough breads that need to be torn with your front teeth, such as hard-crusted French bread. Also to be avoided are foods that need to be chewed for a long period of time. That means no foods harder than scrambled eggs, cottage cheese, soups, soft casseroles, yogurt, and other foods that can be eaten with minimal chewing. If you are worried about adequate nutrition, most meals can be put in a blender and eaten in the soft form. This soft diet will allow the muscles and jaw joint to rest and heal themselves. See appendix for more suggested foods and a diet plan.

3. No Gum

Chewing gum can be very detrimental to the jaw joint and muscles. Vigorously chewing gum even on a healthy jaw joint and muscles can often fatigue the muscles and traumatize the joints so that they become sore from over-

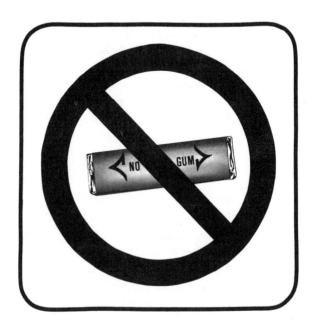

chewing. So, especially if your joint and muscles are sore, avoid chewing gum. If you have a TMJ problem, gum is something that you will probably have to give up for the rest of your life.

4. Relax Your Facial Muscles

Another way to rest your jaw is to relax it. You can say to yourself, "lips at rest, teeth apart, relax my face." This position will put your jaw joint and your muscles in a relaxed position and allow them to heal. Whenever you feel your teeth touching, stop! Take a deep breath. Relax. And repeat, "Lips at rest, teeth apart, relax my face."

5. No Clenching

Your teeth should not touch except when you swallow. Your teeth do not even actually touch when you are chewing food because there is always a small film of food between your teeth. Close your mouth and swallow. You will feel your teeth come together and touch. This is the only time that your teeth should be touching. If you catch yourself with your teeth touching at any other time, this means you are clenching. Your muscles then are putting pressure on your teeth, your jaw joint, and your muscles. This can harm them and make them more painful. Therefore you should attempt to be conscious of whenever your teeth are touching. You should stop, take a deep breath, and say to yourself, "Lips at rest, teeth apart, relax my face." Becoming conscious of clenching will go a long way toward helping heal your jaw and muscles.

6. Yawn Against Pressure

Yawning is another activity that can be detrimental to a sore TMJ. When you yawn, you stretch your muscles and joint ligaments beyond where they normally go. This can tear and injure the joint and muscles. Therefore, you should try to avoid yawning. There are two tricks that you can use to avoid yawning and overopening. One is to make a fist and place it underneath your lower jaw and then yawn against the pressure. This way your fist is supporting your jaw and preventing it from opening too wide. Try it. Make a fist and place it underneath your chin, and try to yawn. You will see that you can still get relief from yawning but prevent your jaw from overopening. Another way to yawn against pressure, especially when your hands are occupied

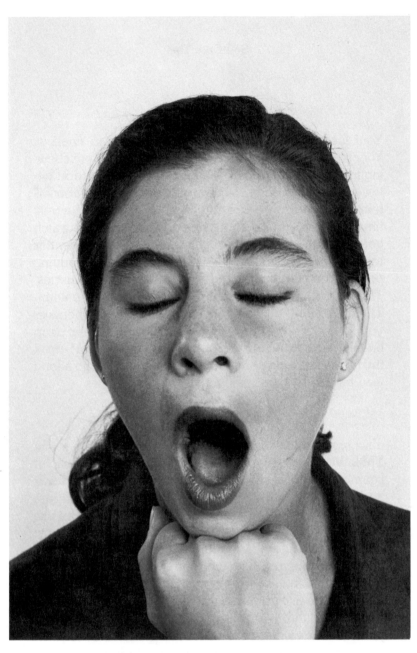

Yawn Against Fist For Support

but you have to yawn, is to place your chin on your chest and yawn. Try it. Bend your head forward so that your chin rests on your chest, then yawn. Your chest is supporting your lower jaw and preventing it from opening too wide.

7. Moist Heat

Heat is another treatment that you can use on sore joints and muscles. Moist heat is much better than dry heat. Moist heat can be applied with a hot, damp towel for 15 to 20 minutes. Heat helps to heal injured muscles and joints by increasing the blood flow, which helps take away the toxins and poisons that have accumulated in injured tissues and brings new healing properties to the area. Heat is also very relaxing to your muscles. Avoid using heat for the first two to three days after a new injury.

8. Ice

Heat should not be applied to new injuries, however. When you sprain your ankle, you do not put heat on it immediately; you put ice on it. The same is true for your TMJ. If you receive a blow to your jaw, immediate treatment with ice is probably much better than heat. Ice reduces the swelling and the pain. Heat would make the swelling worse and probably increase the pain, so with a new injury, avoid heat for the first 48 to 72 hours. Because ice can help reduce the amount of pain, it allows the muscles and joint to be opened and move to their full range. Ice is best for sprains, for muscle pain of long duration such as muscle spasm, and for pain or soreness due to overuse. Ice can be made in a handy form by placing water in a paper or styrofoam cup and freezing it.

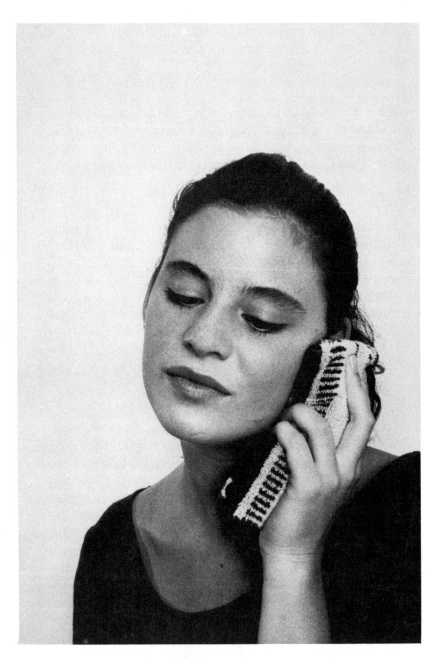

Moist Heat Can Be Applied With Hot Towel

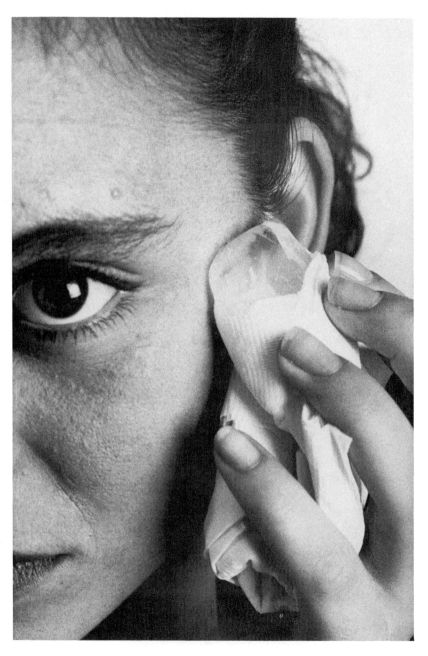

Cold Can Be Applied With Ice

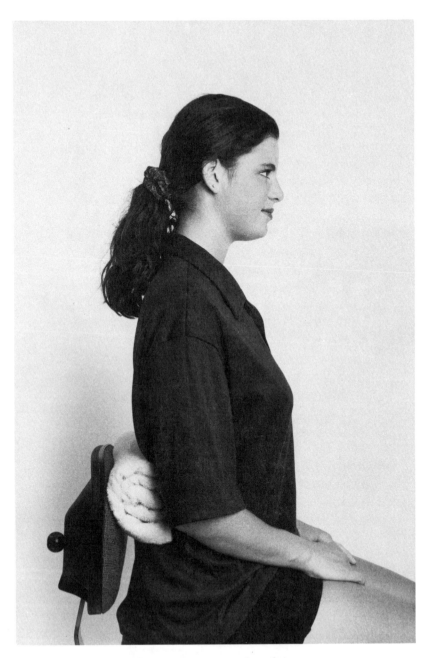

Good Sitting Posture With Towel Providing Lumbar Support

9. Heat and Ice

Heat and ice can also be used in combination to provide relief. First apply heat on the sore or tense muscles for five to ten minutes, and then lightly brush the painful area with ice cubes, placing the ice over the sore areas for two minutes, then heat for two minutes. Repeat this four or five times each session, and finish using cold. This process can be repeated four or five times each day and will give good relief to the pain in your jaw joint and muscles.

10. Good Posture

Posture is also very important in caring for your TMJ and muscle problems. For your muscles to be in balance, your head must sit straight above your shoulders. Your lower back must also be in the correct position so that your head and neck can be in correct position. Learning to sit up straight by using a rolled towel or other lumbar support behind your lower back will help you maintain a good posture. Avoid placing your head forward because this places stress on the muscles of your neck and the muscles of your jaw. Avoid placing your chin down on your chest when studying, reading, or working at a desk. You should avoid leaning on your hand while you are working, reading, or watching TV.

11. Sleeping Position

Posture is also important during sleeping. The best way to sleep as far as your jaw joint and muscles are concerned is on your back. Many people are not able to do this, but if you can, it will allow the muscles of your face, jaw, and neck to be in a more relaxed position. If you sleep on

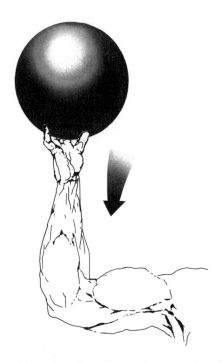

**Bowling Ball Held Straight Over Elbow Does Not Tire Arm Muscles.
Similar to Head Held Straight Over Neck And Shoulders**

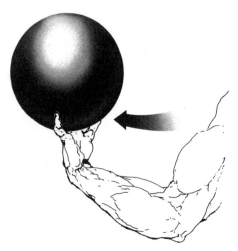

Bowling Ball Not Held Over Elbow Quickly Tires And Strains Muscles

your side with either an arm or a hard pillow under your jaw, your jaw can be pushed far to one side, putting a strain on your TMJ and muscles. Therefore, even if you aren't comfortable sleeping on your back, you need to be conscious of the position of your jaw while you sleep and try to get out of the habit of sleeping in positions that may put stress on it.

12. Jaw Exercise

You can do several simple jaw exercises to help strengthen and retrain your jaw muscles. A simple exercise is to stand in front of a mirror, place the tip of your tongue on the roof of your mouth just behind your front teeth. Keep the tip of the tongue there and slowly open and close your mouth, making sure it opens and closes in a straight line. Repeat this ten times in the morning and ten times at night.

Another exercise is to open and close your mouth ten times, using your thumb and forefinger on your chin to apply light backward pressure.

13. Exercise

A regular program of exercise can make you feel much better, both physically and emotionally. Exercise helps to counteract the effects of stress and it makes you feel better about yourself. It gets the muscles and organs of your body working in a healthier way. Exercise has been shown to release chemicals called endorphins into your bloodstream that make you feel better and also can help counter the effects of pain. Endorphins are thought to be natural opiates and have a beneficial effect on how you feel about yourself. In fact, some psychiatrists and psychologists

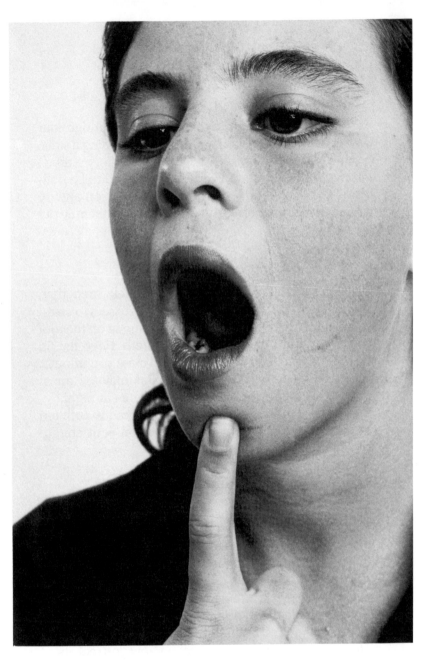

**Opening And Closing Against Finger Pressure
Is Good Exercise For TMJ**

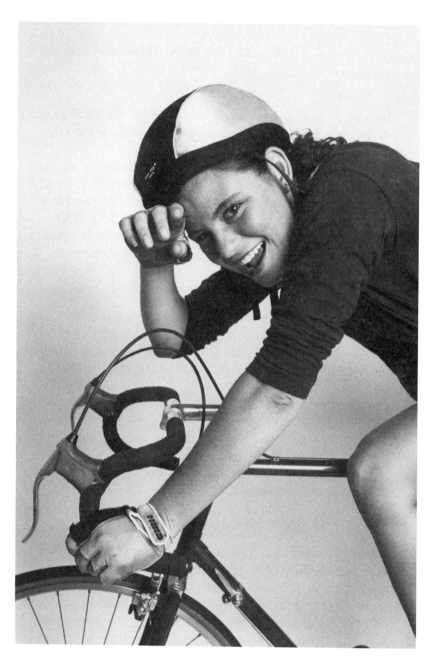

Exercise

believe that regular exercise can help in the treatment of anxiety and depression as well as other emotional problems.

A regular exercise program does not have to be running 10 miles a day or taking high-energy aerobics. It just needs to be something that is comfortable to you and that you can do regularly for 15 or 20 minutes four times a week. A regular exercise program can be as simple as taking a brisk 20-minute walk at least four times a week.

14. Acupressure

Acupressure is using pressure on acupuncture points to get relief and healing. One point that is excellent for relief of headaches and jaw pain is located between the thumb and first finger. Put your thumb and first finger together and follow the crease to the end, then go to the highest point on the muscle towards the first finger. That is the acupuncture point Hoku. Now firmly press with the point of a finger on that point until you feel an aching or uncomfortable feeling. Then gently press on that area for five minutes. Often you will experience a dramatic relief of pain in your head and jaw.

15. Over-the-Counter Medications

If you still have pain in your jaw and muscles, then you can take medication to relieve the pain. There are many over-the-counter medications you can take for pain, but with TMJ problems, medications not only lessen pain but also reduce inflammation in the joint and muscles. The over-the-counter medications that can do both are those that have aspirin or ibuprofen in them. In order to reduce

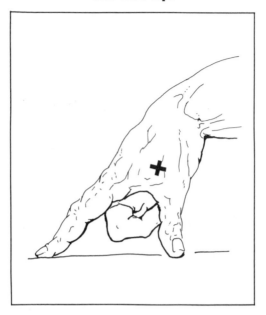

**Acupuncture Point Hoku Located Between Thumb And Forefinger.
Pressure Massage On This Point Provides Relief For Jaw And Head Pain**

inflammation, aspirin must be taken in large doses, that is, two tablets four times a day in order to get a high enough blood level. Just taking one or two aspirin tablets will relieve the pain but will not have a long-term effect in reducing the inflammation in the joint or muscle that is causing the pain. Likewise, ibuprofen (or Motrin) also needs to be taken four times a day in order to build up a blood level that will sustain the anti-inflammatory effects as well as the pain-fighting effects.

Tylenol, the brand name for the chemical acetaminophen, is a good over-the-counter pain reliever but has little or no anti-inflammatory effects. Therefore it is not the best medication to use in cases of temporomandibular joint pain.

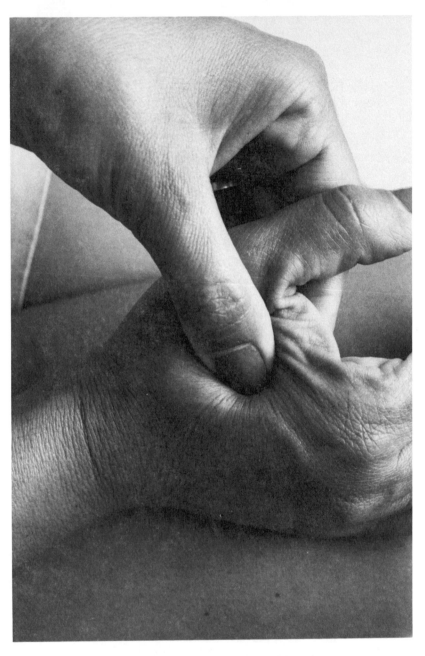

**Acupressure Between Thumb And Forefinger
Can Provide Relief For Jaw Pain**

Over-the-counter medications should not be taken for more than a couple of weeks without discussing the problems with your doctor. All medications have side effects, and long-term use increases the side effects. The goal is to be pain free without medication, so if you need medication, it should be taken for a limited period of time only. If you find you need to take medication on a more than short-term basis, you should talk with your doctor or dentist about a different treatment plan or a different medication that will give more permanent solution to your problem.

16. Yoga and Meditation

Meditation, of which yoga is one form, helps by relaxing the body and counteracting many of the characteristics of stress reactions. Meditative practices date back over 2,000 years. As with acupuncture, there is a long history of therapeutic claims to meditative practices. There are claims of curing or alleviating conditions such as constipation, gas pains, sunken chest, round shoulders, nasal drip, fallen arches, sciatica, bursitis, menstrual disorders, aching back, and aching psyche.

Studies have been done in modern Western medicine to test these claims. These studies have shown that major changes occur during meditation, such as slowing of breath and heart rate, decrease in oxygen consumption, lowering of blood pressure, decrease in skin conductivity, and changes in the electric currents to the brain. The interesting thing about all these responses is that they are the opposite of the traditional fight-or-flight response of the stress reaction. Therefore, meditative techniques have been tried and

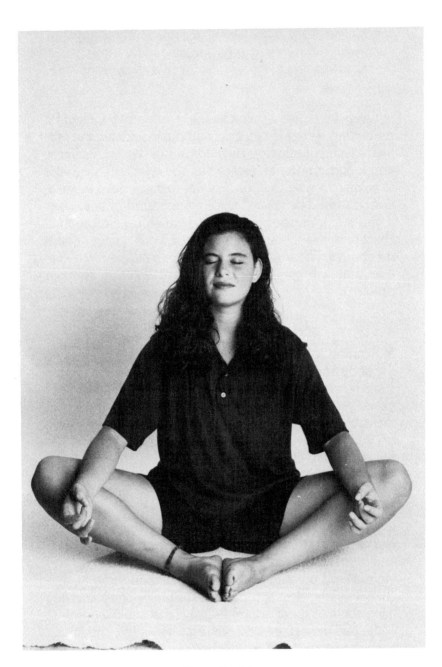

Yoga Position

tested as a method to counteract the harmful effects of stress. Most of these studies have shown positive results.

Yoga is one of the most publicized meditative techniques in this country. It combines exercises with meditation to bring about a relaxed state. It is aimed at integrating the body and the mind.

The stretching exercises of yoga are particularly helpful in relieving nervous tension, since all stretching is inherently tranquilizing. Most of us have noticed that animals, upon rising, will stretch. Not only dogs and cats but also zoo animals, unless they are alarmed, will stretch right after they awake. Humans naturally stretch too. When we awake from a particularly restful sleep, the first thing we do is stretch.

In yoga, tensing exercises, that is, contracting and strengthening the muscles, are used to teach breath control. They also can help tense people relax, since controlled tension often seems to lead to a controlled letting go.

Bends and twists increase mobility of limbs, stretching of ligaments, lubrication of joints, and creating a supple, flexible spine. Gentle flowing motions combined with rhythmic breathing can improve circulation and coordination. All this takes concentration, and the focus of attention inside one's self helps the mind control the body.

Meditation is only one part of an individual's total behavior. It is not a miracle cure for everything that is wrong with a person. Even though meditation can have a very positive effect upon one's entire life, it cannot constitute an entire treatment program for TMJ problems. Its main value for people with TMJ problems is its effect in reversing stress.

There are many advertisements in local magazines and other publications for classes in various types of yoga and meditation. Many educational networks, schools, and recreational centers offer classes in both meditation and yoga.

17. Good Nutrition

In general, people with TMJ problems need to have a generally healthy diet so that their body can heal and repair itself. A healthy diet means a person is physically in a healthier state, which usually leads to healthy state of mind as well. Good general physical health goes hand in hand with good general emotional health.

Vitamins and minerals are also important for the healing and repair of muscles. Vitamin B1 (thiamine), Vitamin B6, or pyridoxide, and Vitamin B12 are the important B vitamins that are involved in muscle metabolism and muscle repair. Vitamin C (ascorbic acid) is also important in muscle healing, especially in terms of strengthening capillaries and healing of muscle tissue.

You should try to eat a balanced diet that includes foods that will provide the necessary requirements for vitamins and minerals. If you do this, there is no need to take additional vitamins. If for some reason you are unable to get a balanced diet, then vitamin and mineral supplements are a good idea.

Minerals and their functions:

1. Calcium, nitrogen and sulfur are needed for the formation of protein.
2. Potassium is necessary for the proper functioning of nerves and the heart.

3. Cobalt has to be present in order for Vitamin B-12 to work.
4. Zinc is utilized as part of insulin molecule that is necessary to absorb sugar.
5. Minerals such as manganese, copper, cobalt, iodine, zinc, magnesium and phosphorous are needed for both physical and mental energy.
6. Calcium and phosphorous are essential for strong bones and teeth.

Several groups of people have much higher requirements for vitamins and minerals than normal. Among these are the pregnant women, the elderly, substance abusers, and the poor and homeless. These groups often do not get a high enough level of vitamins for optimum healing to take place.

In addition, alcohol, tobacco and caffeine all have detrimental effects on the intake of vitamins. Alcohol abuse can lead to reduced intake of vitamins as well as destruction of the liver, which is necessary for healing. Tobacco smoking markedly increases the need for Vitamin C. Caffeine in excess of two or three cups a day can cause aggravation of muscle trigger points.

18. Massage

Massage is an excellent way to reduce muscle soreness and muscle tension. If your TMJ problem includes sore muscles, massage of those muscles is an excellent method of improving the soreness. This massage can be by a person trained in massage, by a friend, or by yourself.

There are many different types of massage — very light

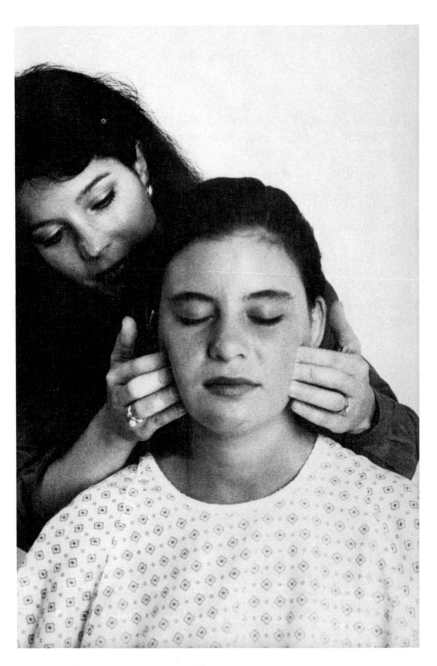

Massage

massage, deep massage, hard massage, vibrating massage — and each type has a specific effect. Another type of massage, called acupressure, is a combination of massage and acupuncture and utilizes massage of acupuncture points (*see page 96*). Different people are helped by different types of massage, and in fact, different problems are helped by different types of massage.

Trigger points are tender spots in the muscle that refer pain to other areas. Deep massage is very helpful. Deep massage needs to be done many times in a repetitive motion until the nodules, or trigger points, disappear. This often relieves the local tenderness and the referred pain that the trigger point in the muscle was causing.

Some people are helped by a firm, heavy, friction type of massage. Others find a stroking or kneading type of massage more effective, and still others find that a light stroking massage is helpful. Each person needs to experiment to find out which type of massage is best for their specific need.

Massage works in many different ways: it relieves the soreness in the specific muscle or muscles, and it causes a general relaxation of the body, which tends to relax the muscles and relieve tension and stress. It increases the circulation in muscles and breaks up adhesions. For these reasons, it is very helpful for many patients.

19. Athletic Mouthguard

You can use an athletic mouthguard instead of a splint (*see page 113*), but there are several disadvantages. A mouthguard is very bulky and has to be formed by placing it in hot water and biting into it. Since a mouthguard is so bulky, it is usually uncomfortable to wear over long periods of time. Many people have difficulty sleeping with an athletic mouthguard. Because mouthguards are made out of soft, rubbery material, you may tend to bite into the mouthguard and use your muscles even more. The one big advantage is that mouthguards are very cheap and readily available. The bottom line is that you can use a mouthguard, but if your problems in any way get worse or do not improve, you should discontinue wearing it. If worn for long periods of time, a mouthguard can act as an orthodontic appliance and move teeth, so long-term wear should be discouraged. You should consult your dentist after one month to be sure there are no dental problems.

20. Avoid Long Dental Appointments

Dental appointments that require you to keep your mouth open for more than thirty minutes can strain your muscles and activate a problem. The stress of undergoing dental treatment can also make your muscles very tense. If you undergo dental treatment, explain to your dentist that you have a TMJ problem and that you need to stop and rest every five to ten minutes for one minute. This will greatly reduce the strain on your muscles and joint. You can schedule shorter appointments and visit your dentist more frequently.

Extraction of teeth can also be very detrimental to your TMJ if heavy force is applied. Again, inform your dentist and he or she may be able to use special techniques such as sectioning or cutting the tooth into pieces so it may be removed easily without the use of much force.

Some dentists have patients use a bite block, a rubber wedge that is inserted between the back teeth to help them

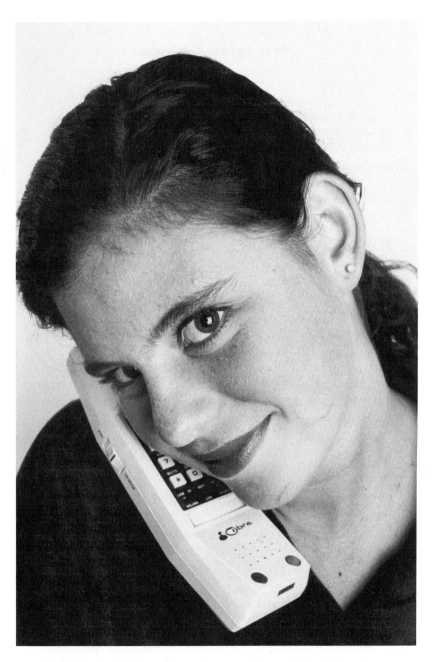

Cradling Telephone Can Cause Jaw And Neck Problems

keep the mouth wide open. If you have a TMJ problem, inform your dentist to use care in not stretching your mouth too far open as this can aggravate your condition and cause damage and pain. Again, shorter appointments are much better than long ones.

21. Avoid General Anesthesia

Another source of injury to your TMJ can be caused by general anesthetics administered for surgery. When you are put to sleep the anesthesiologist places a tube into your mouth and down into the trachea, which leads to the lungs. In doing this, the jaw can be opened too wide, tearing or straining the joint. Your muscles are completely relaxed at this time and offer little protection to the jaw being strained. Let your doctor know you have a TMJ problem so he or she can either be extra careful, or use a technique that places the tube through the nose into the trachea. This procedure is called nasotracheal intubation.

22. Telephone Use

The telephone is, of course, a common device that everyone uses. It can be harmful to your TMJ and muscles if you cradle it between your jaw and shoulder without using your hands. This position is bad posture for both your neck and jaw and can cause muscle and joint problems. Avoid using that position for the telephone.

If Your Jaw Locks Open

When the jaw opens too wide, especially during a yawn, it can slip out of place and lock in a forward position outside the joint. This can be very painful and uncomfortable.

If this happens, you need to try to get your jaw to go back into place. If you are unable to do this after trying for a few minutes, ask a friend or neighbor to help you by pressing downward and backward with his or her thumbs inside your mouth but outside your back teeth (so that if your jaw snaps closed, you won't bite the thumbs). You may be unable to speak, so you may have to write a note describing what to do. You can apply ice to your jaw and often that will help get it back into place.

If your jaw cannot be corrected quickly, you should see a dentist immediately or go to an emergency room. There, somebody will be able to place your jaw back into position. If the muscles go into spasm, you may need to be given an anesthetic to relax them before the jaw can be placed back into the proper position.

After the jaw is back into position, you will need to place ice over the joints to reduce swelling and pain. Aspirin is also helpful for pain and reduction of inflammation in the joint. You should start on a soft diet so that your jaw can rest and heal. You then need to make an appointment with either your doctor or dentist to have the problem evaluated.

If You Can't Open Your Mouth

There are two reasons TMJ disorders can prevent you from opening your mouth. The first one is muscle spasm. The muscles can go into spasm and contract and thus limit the amount that you can open your mouth. This can happen either because of tension or stress of the muscle or because of trauma, such as an accident.

The second reason is that the disc or pad in the joint can be displaced and act as a block when you try to open your mouth. When the disc has been displaced, you will be able to open your mouth usually only about one to one and a half fingers wide. This is because the disc is out in front of the jawbone and acts as a block to further opening.

You can start immediate treatment yourself by taking aspirin for the pain, placing ice over your jaw joints and sore muscles, and gently opening your mouth as wide as you can without pain.

Both muscle spasm and displaced disc are treatable by physical therapy. You may also need other treatments, such as medications and a splint.

Herbal Medicines That Can Help

Some people are inclined to use natural or herbal remedies rather than drugs. Although prescription drugs are packaged in many different forms and colors, and we tend to think of them as chemicals, many doctors' prescriptions contain drugs from natural plant sources. The most famous drug from plants is digitalis, which is used for heart failure. It increases the force of contraction of the heart muscle. It comes from the leaves of the foxglove or digitalis plant.

So even though the line between drugs and natural herbs is clouded, many natural remedies can be of help.

Many herbal teas such as peppermint, spearmint, camomile, rose hips, alfalfa, angelica, lemon verbena, sage, thyme, clover and anise seed can have a very calming effect on one's psyche. And the very act of relaxing with a hot cup of tea can in itself provide a calming effect, and reduce the stress of the day. When these teas contain herbs that have a chemical effect, they act like medicines. Below are examples of some herbal remedies.

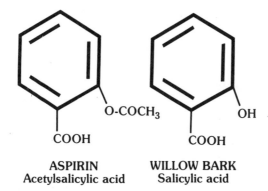

ASPIRIN
Acetylsalicylic acid

WILLOW BARK
Salicylic acid

1. **Willow bark tea.** Boil the inner root bark from any of the willows and make a strong tea. Willow bark contains salicylic acid, which is chemically related to aspirin. It is good for reducing inflammation and fevers and for the relief of pain.
2. **Wintergreen.** Oil of wintergreen contains methyl salicylate, which is closely related to aspirin and is used to help body aches and pains, including sore joints. It can be used by soaking gauze in wintergreen and applying it to sore joints or muscles. It also can be used by drinking a tea prepared from the leaves.
3. **Watercress.** Using Watercress as a soup or tea, or eating the plant raw (as in a salad) will provide relief from pain and swelling. It contains salicylic acid.
4. **Spikenoud.** A poultice prepared from the pulverized root can be applied to sore joints and muscles for relief. It contains a chemical called aralin.

5. **Pennyroyal.** The leaves can be made into a tea that is good for headaches.

6. **Pokeweed.** A tea made from the boiled berries of pokeweed is said to provide relief from sore joints.

7. **Wild Black Cherry.** The bark is soaked in warm water and is drunk as a sedative. This can provide relief from both stress and pain.

8. **Hops.** Hops are used in brewing beer to add bitterness and to act as a preservative. Hops contain a chemical called lupulin, which is a sedative and hypnotic drug. A tea made from the fruiting bodies can have a profound calming effect.

CHAPTER 8

DENTAL TREATMENTS FOR TMJ

Dentists, being experts of the teeth and jaws, have become the specialists who know the most about treating TMJ disorders. Dentists use splints, medications, and surgery as the most accepted treatments for TMJ disorders.

Splints

A splint (also called an orthotic) is often of great help to people who have TMJ problems. Splints are usually clear plastic appliances that fit in the mouth and cover either the top teeth or the bottom teeth. A splint keeps the teeth apart and reduces the effects of bruxism on the teeth, and joint, and muscles. A splint helps relax the jaw muscles by opening them up and making them longer and, because you hit the splint when you clench your teeth, it makes you aware that you are putting your muscles under

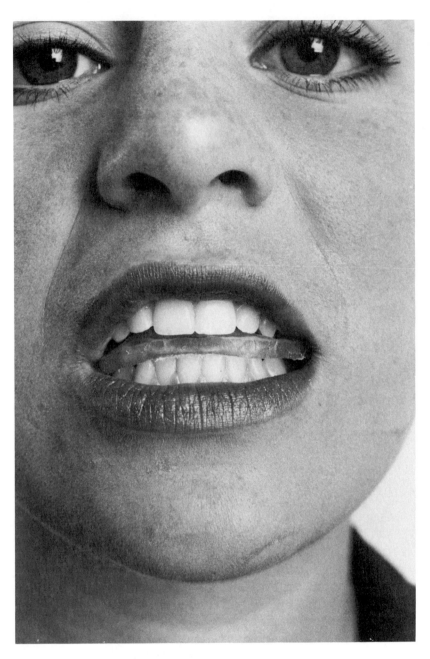

Splints (Orthotics) Separate Teeth

114

tension. The splint thus helps break the habit of clenching your jaw muscles. The third way that a splint works is to place your jaw joint in a different position, which can help it heal by reducing the pressure on it.

There are basically three types of splints. The first type is a splint to prevent grinding the teeth. This is called a bruxism splint, or night guard. It is normally worn at night to protect the teeth from being worn down and to more evenly distribute the forces in the jaw muscles and joints. Many dentists used to think that these bruxism splints helped prevent people from grinding their teeth, but recent research shows that this is not true. People will still brux, but they will be doing it on the splint instead of on their teeth. The splint also protects the teeth from the harmful effects of grinding, that is, from wearing them down, cracking them, breaking fillings, and making them sensitive.

Another type of splint is a stabilizing splint. This splint is worn 24 hours a day and helps place the muscles and joints in a better position so that they are more relaxed and under less pressure and therefore healing can take place. The stabilizing splint also reduces the effects of bruxism, as does the night guard or bruxism splint. Another reason the stabilizing splint is effective is that you must eat soft foods, which reduces the amount of trauma to the jaw muscles and enables them to heal.

The third type of splint is a repositioning splint. This splint is usually used when one or both of the discs in the jaw joint has been torn and displaced and it is necessary to reposition the jaw to promote healing of the tissues. This type of splint is also worn both day and night and works in the same ways that the other two splints work.

How Long Will I Need To Wear The Splint?

If you need a splint for bruxism, you may have to wear it at night for as long as you grind your teeth. If the splint is needed to reposition your jaw to allow for healing of the displaced disc in the joint, you may only have to wear it for a few weeks or months. In short, how long you have to wear the splints depends on your injury and how well you comply with the instructions about wearing the splint.

Most people wear their splints until their jaw and muscles have healed and they no longer have any pain. You will probably not have to wear the splint longer than six months unless your doctor feels that you need it to protect you from grinding your teeth at night. Many people do continue to wear their splints at night or only when their jaw joints and muscles are acting up again. When they feel tenderness or pain over their jaw muscles or joints, they wear their splint for a few days or weeks, until the symptoms have subsided.

Dental Checkups

You need to have your progress monitored on a regular basis to see how your symptoms are responding to the treatment. Most TMJ splints will also need to be periodically adjusted. As the joint and muscles heal, your bite will change and your teeth will meet differently on the splint. If your splint is a repositioning one, you will probably need to have it adjusted periodically to change the position back to your original one as healing progresses. The only splint that does not need to be adjusted is the one worn to protect your teeth from the effects of grinding, or bruxism. You need to have this kind of splint checked only when there are problems with it or when you go for your regular checkups.

In a small number of cases the healing that takes place after wearing a splint places the jaw in a new, comfortable position, but the teeth may not meet correctly and it may not be possible to chew or eat or be without pain unless you are wearing the splint. In these cases, either you will have to wear a splint for the rest of your life or your teeth will have to be moved into the new position so that you can eat and chew comfortably without the splint. If the teeth need to be moved only slightly, they can be selectively ground so that they meet in a new position. If the distance is greater, then you may need crowns or caps so that your teeth can meet in the new position, or orthodontics or braces can move your teeth into the new position. If the discrepancy is very great, your teeth or jaws may need to be moved by surgery. But such cases are, fortunately, very rare, and most people can find relief of their symptoms without extensive dental work. This dental work is not done as a treatment for your TMJ symptoms. In fact, it should not be done until your symptoms have gone. Then it should be done for dental reasons such as to make you better able to chew and eat.

Difficulties Wearing A Splint

Because they are made of clear plastic, splints usually do not create too much of a problem with appearance. Most people have more difficulty adjusting to the feel of the splint, to something foreign inside the mouth that makes it difficult to talk. Most patients will get used to a splint in one to two weeks if they wear it all the time. The tongue adjusts to the feeling of the plastic shield in the mouth, and speech usually becomes normal in about a week. Eating is more difficult, however, and if you are wearing a splint 24 hours a day, you will need to stick to a soft diet. You will not be able to chew hard foods, but this is something that you want to avoid anyway when you are trying to allow your joint and muscles to heal.

Cleaning And Maintaining Your Splint

Your splint must be cleaned every time you brush your teeth. Take your splint out and use your toothbrush to clean it inside and out. You can keep your splint in a container with water if you do not wear it during the day. Soaking it once in a while in a denture cleanser or placing a teaspoon of vinegar in the water will help clean and freshen the splint. Your splint will wear as you use it so you should inspect it for cracks and other signs of wear. If you notice cracks in the splint, take it to the dentist to be repaired. Any rubbing on the soft parts of your mouth can cause blisters or sore spots, and this is another sign that the splint should be adjusted by your dentist. Your splint should be comfortable and not cause any pain or discomfort.

Trigger Point Therapy

Trigger point therapy is performed by physicians and dentists for myofascial pain. Trigger points are small, painful knots located in various muscles of the body that produce referred pain. The pain is felt in a part of the body at a distance from the actual painful knot. These areas can be injected with a small amount of local anesthetic. This will provide dramatic relief of the referred pain that is felt somewhere else. This can be very instructional for both the patient and the doctor and can help arrive at a clear diagnosis.

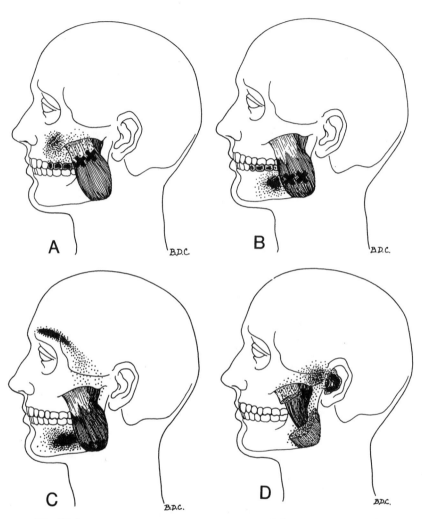

The X's locate trigger points in various parts of the masseter muscle. *Solid* shows essential referred pain zones, and the *stippled areas* are spillover pain zones. A, superficial layer, upper section. B, superficial layer, mid-belly. C, lower portion. D, deep layer, upper part — just below the temporomandibular joint. © Janet G. Travell, M.D., *Myofascial Pain and Dysfunction: The Trigger Point Manual,* published by Williams and Wilkins.

119

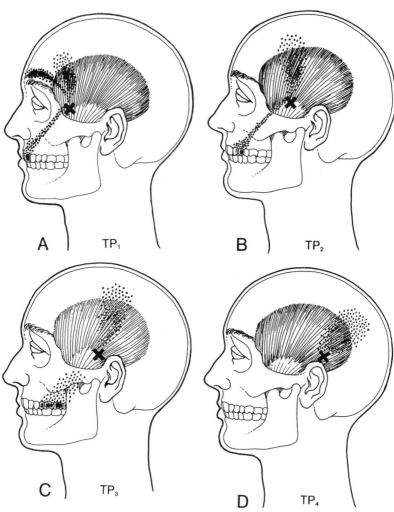

Referred pain patterns from trigger points (X's) in the left temporalis muscle (essential zones *solid,* spillover zones *stippled*). A, anterior "spokes" of pain arising from the anterior fibers (trigger point one region). B and C, middle "spokes" (trigger point two and trigger point three regions). D, posterior supra-auricular "spoke" (trigger point four region). © Janet G. Travell, M.D., *Myofascial Pain and Dysfunction: The Trigger Point Manual,* published by Williams and Wilkins.

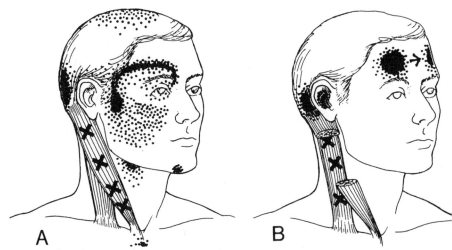

Referred pain patterns (*solid lines* show essential zones and *stippling* shows the spillover areas) with location corresponding trigger points (X's) in the right sternocleidomastoid muscle. A, the sternal (superficial) division. B, the clavicular (deep) division. © Janet G. Travell, M.D., *Myofascial Pain and Dysfunction: The Trigger Point Manual,* published by Williams and Wilkins.

Studies have found that these trigger points do not have to be injected with local anesthetic. Salt water will also work and in some cases just the needling will work. Massage of these trigger points will also help alleviate them. Spray and stretch techniques, where a coolant is sprayed on the skin and then the muscle is gently stretched, also work to stop the pain.

Prescription Medications

R Your doctor or dentist can prescribe a variety of medications depending on what your problem is and how you respond to medications.

Aspirin may be the drug that your dentist will recommend for you. Even though a prescription is not needed for aspirin, your dentist may recommend that you take aspirin in higher doses than normal. Aspirin acts as a painkiller and an anti-inflammatory agent at levels of two to three grams per day. Taking aspirin in high doses such as these needs to be followed by a doctor because you may get side effects, such as ringing in the ears, and the amount of the drug may need to be reduced. You should always take aspirin with food or juice to reduce the irritation to the stomach.

Your dentist may prescribe ibuprofen in doses that you can only get by prescription. It is supplied as tablets in 400, 600, 800 milligrams. It should be prescribed for at least ten days to determine if it is going to be effective. Like aspirin, it should be taken with food or juice to reduce the amount of irritation to the stomach lining. Anyone one with stomach ulcers should not take aspirin or ibuprofen, or probably any drugs, without carefully talking it over with their doctor.

Naprosyn, or naproxen, is an anti-inflammatory drug similar to Motrin or ibuprofen. It is supplied as tablets in 250, 375, or 500 milligrams. The usual dosage is 375 milligrams twice a day with food or juice.

Feldene, also known as piroxicam, is supplied in 10 and 20 milligram capsules, and the dosage is one 20-milligram capsule per day taken with food. The advantage of feldene is that you only need to take one capsule per day. The disadvantage is that it can be very irritating to the stomach lining. It also has other toxic side effects, and 30 percent of patients are said to experience some side effects. You need to monitor the taking of feldene very closely and report any side effects to your doctor.

This completes the list of the most commonly used anti-

DRUG CHART

General Category	Brand Name	Chemical Name	Main Actions	Main Side Effects
Painkiller	Aspirin, Anacin, Bufferin, Ascriptin, Cope, Empirin	Acetylsalicylic acid	reduces pain reduces fever reduces inflammation	irritates stomach
Painkiller	Tylenol Datril, Anacin II	acetaminophen	reduces pain reduces fever	none
Anti-inflammatory	Motrin, Advil	ibuprofen	reduces pain reduces inflammation	irritates stomach
Anti-inflammatory	Naprosyn	naproxen	reduces pain reduces inflammation	irritates stomach
Anti-inflammatory	Feldene	piroxicam	reduces pain reduces inflammation	irritates stomach
Anti-depressant	Elavil	amitriptyline	reduces pain reduces depression	loss of energy dry mouth
Anti-depressant	Tofranil	imipramine	reduces pain reduces depression	loss of energy dry mouth
Minor tranquilizer	Valium	diazepam	reduces tension and anxiety	addiction or dependence drowsiness
Major tranquilizer	Thorazine	chlorpromazine	severe psychiatric states chronic pain	drowsiness mood depression
Major tranquilizer	Compazine	prochlorperazine	severe psychiatric states chronic pain	drowsiness mood depression

inflammatory medications. They all have actions that help reduce pain and help reduce the inflammation in the joints and muscles that cause pain.

Valium, or diazepam, is a mood-altering drug that is used to reduce anxiety and tension. Prolonged use of Valium can result in a dependence or addiction to it. Therefore it should be used only for short-term or periodic therapy. Because it can reduce stress or anxiety, Valium has been shown to be useful in reducing bruxism, or night grinding. But it should be taken for bruxism only during times of stress. Since Valium is addicting and the answer to dealing with stress is not with drugs, it should be taken for only a very short time. If Valium is taken over a prolonged period, a significant depression of mood can result. Valium should not be taken with alcohol, because the effect of the combination of Valium and alcohol enhances the danger of a toxic reaction. For various reasons Valium is one of the most abused drugs in this country and therefore its casual use should be discouraged. However, for specific occasions and for limited periods of time, it may be very helpful.

Anti-depressants, such as Elavil, Sinequan, Tofranil, and Aventyl are used in large doses for the relief of symptoms of depression, but they can cause many side effects, including dry mouth, drowsiness, blurred vision, tingling fingers, and changes in blood pressure. Recent studies have shown that anti-depressants used in much lower doses are good pain relievers for TMJ and other pain. Anti-depressants in low doses have also been shown to reduce bruxism, or night grinding, which is one of the causes of muscle and joint soreness. Taking a low dose of an anti-depressant drug once a day just before bedtime reduces some of the side effects because they are less noticeable during the night.

One of the reasons medications work is the placebo effect. A placebo, or sugar pill, has no scientifically known method of action. Yet placebos work for about 40 percent of the people who take them. That means that out of a group of 100 people, 40 will experience at least some improvement by taking a sugar pill. This is called the placebo response, and it may be related to many different things. Some people believe that a placebo works because a doctor tells you that it will be good for you and you believe that it will. This is similar to the power of suggestion. Other people believe that taking a placebo induces a form of self-hypnosis or that simply desire to improve will cause an improvement. One theory is that self-hypnosis or the desire to improve releases endorphins, the naturally occurring painkillers in one's body. At any rate, any medication has a placebo effect. But many medications also have an effect that is much greater than a placebo effect.

It is important to remember that every drug is used for a specific purpose and with a specific goal in mind. You need to understand what the purpose and the goal are, because you do not want to be taking medications forever. The goal is alleviation of the pain while your TMJ heals.

Dental Work

Dental treatment as a cure for TMJ problems has given dentistry a bad name. An article in Forbes (August 1984) states:

> Overtreatment is widespread with regard to what
> dentists call temporomandibular joint syndrome. . . .
> From coast to coast, unethical dentists treat gullible pa-

tients for TMJ syndrome with all manner of procedures ranging from splints to fillings to major surgery, which can cost over $10,000. . . . This money can easily make a struggling dentist solvent. And don't think word about the TMJ hasn't gotten around. A 1981 advertisement by Long Island University's Institute for Continuing Education in the Journal of the American Dental Association featured the headline: How to increase, revitalize and inflation proof your practice through TMJ.

For many years the dental profession thought that bad bites, or malocclusions, caused TMJ problems, but research studies have shown that people with bad bites won't show any higher incidence of TMJ problems than people with normal bites. It also used to be thought that bad bites caused bruxism, or grinding of the teeth at night. But research has also shown that this is not so. Research subjects were given crowns that created a bad bite, and the activity of their jaw muscles was measured at night with electrodes; the results showed that these people did not brux any more with artificially created bad bites than they did without them. As a result of all this research, it is generally the understanding today that bad bites do not cause TMJ problems.

Nevertheless, many dentists are still treating TMJ problems by grinding the teeth, placing crowns on the teeth, bonding teeth, or moving the teeth through orthodontics or through jaw surgery. In most cases, this kind of dental work should not be done unless a person needs crowns or orthodontics to make their bite look better, make their teeth easier to keep clean and less susceptible to decay, or allow them to chew better.

In my opinion, the reason that bad bites do not often

cause problems is that the body is able to adapt to various changes over time. A bad bite is something that a person is born with or that develops gradually. It is not something that hits all of a sudden. Your body, your muscles, your bones, your TMJ all adapt to a gradual change in your bite and you are able to cope with it. Unless your bite changes dramatically over a short period of time, because of a broken jaw, or a new bridge or crown that does not fit, or extraction of back teeth, it usually does not cause TMJ problems.

As we previously discussed, however, after treatment of your TMJ problem with a splint, dental work may be necessary so that you can chew better, your teeth will meet in a more stable position with your jaw joint, and your muscles will be in balance in the new position created by the splint. Dental work is not necessarily a treatment or cure for your TMJ problem but, rather, a way to rebuild your mouth so that you will be able to chew better in the new position in which your jaw has healed.

Surgery

A Deformed Jaw

Joan had headaches, earaches, and pain when she chewed hard food. Her complaint started about a month before she came to see me, at a time when she had been under a lot of stress because of examinations and schoolwork. I examined her and found both of her temporomandibular joints to be very sore, as were her muscles in the temple and cheek area.

I noted that one side of her face was larger than

the other side. Also, her bite was off on one side, and the teeth slanted towards the side that was not as well developed. An x-ray showed that the condyle or part of her lower jaw that fits into the socket had not developed. It was very small when compared to the condyle on the other side of her jaw. Joan was also concerned about having her teeth straightened and correcting the facial deformity that she had. She started on a program of home care for her temporomandibular joint problem. She started on a soft diet, used heat and ice for the sore muscles and was taking aspirin for the pain and inflammation. She was taught how to keep her teeth apart and relax her facial muscles and was shown how that when she was under stress, she would clench her teeth. She was instructed to try to work on lessening the amount of clenching of her teeth and to try to recognize the stress that she was under and do some simple things to try to alleviate the stress. Within a month her symptoms of headaches, earaches, and inability to chew hard foods had disappeared and she had no further complaints with her jaw. She was then referred to an oral surgeon who developed a plan for surgically correcting her facial deformity and bad bite with the help of an orthodontist. This was being done not to treat her TMJ problem but her facial deformity, which affected her appearance, and her crowded teeth, which also affected her appearance and gave her an unstable bite.

Surgery is probably used in less than 5 percent of all TMJ problems. It is a treatment of last resort, to be used when other, more conservative approaches have been tried and have not been successful. TMJ surgery is like back surgery in that back surgery used to be the number-one approach for severe back problems, but now most back problems can be managed with other treatments — physical therapy, traction, medication, and exercise. In the same way, 95 percent of all TMJ problems can be corrected by physical therapy, splint therapy, exercises, medications, and other, more conservative, approaches.

For cases that do not improve and that have evidence of damage that can be corrected surgically, surgery can be helpful. Conditions that may require surgery are tumors, severe dislocations, dislocated discs, and conditions where the jaw is locked and unable to be opened.

There are three types of surgery. One is the traditional surgery to the joint, where an incision is made over the joint and the joint is surgically opened up. This type of open joint surgery has certain risks, one being nerve damage, which can cause facial paralysis. However, this is the only approach that can be used if any major work is to be done inside the joint.

The second type of surgery is called microscopic surgery. It is a form of open joint surgery where an incision about one inch long is made just in front of the ear. The TMJ is opened up and reconstructed using a microscope and special fiber optic lighting that allows the surgeon to perform detailed procedures under magnification.

The third type of surgery is arthroscopic surgery. This type of surgery is most common in the knee. A tiny tube is inserted into a small incision, through which the surgeon can look into the joint. The surgeon can insert small surgical instruments through this tube and remove scar

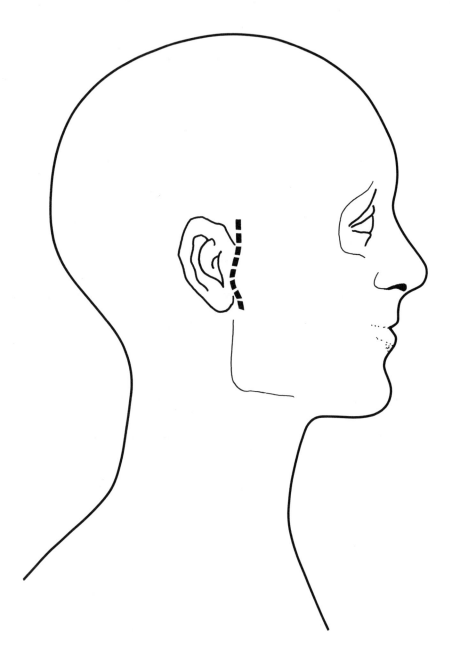

Typical Incision For TMJ Open Joint Surgery
About One To Two Inches Long, Just In Front Of Ear

130

tissue and irrigate and flush out the joint. This is often all that is necessary to have a successful surgery.

Surgery can be helpful for elimination of pain and restoration of function in some cases. But it should be used only where there is evidence of some disorder that can be surgically corrected and conservative treatment has failed. It should not be used to prevent pain or further disease. It also should not be used in any of the various types of arthritis.

Surgery also needs to be followed by physical therapy, medications, and exercises in order to be successful.

Notes

CHAPTER 9

TREATMENT BY OTHER HEALTH CARE PROVIDERS

TMJ disorders can be helped by many different health care providers. Some clinics have a team approach where specialists in many different fields will all have input into the treatment of one patient. In other settings this is done by referral.

Physical Therapy

Many people can completely manage their TMJ problems with nothing more than physical therapy. Physical therapists, with their extensive knowledge of the muscles, bones, and joints, play an important role in educating, managing, and treating TMJ problems. Your physical therapist will evaluate you for muscle tension and tenderness, stress in your muscles, the functioning of your joints and, very importantly, your posture, or relationship

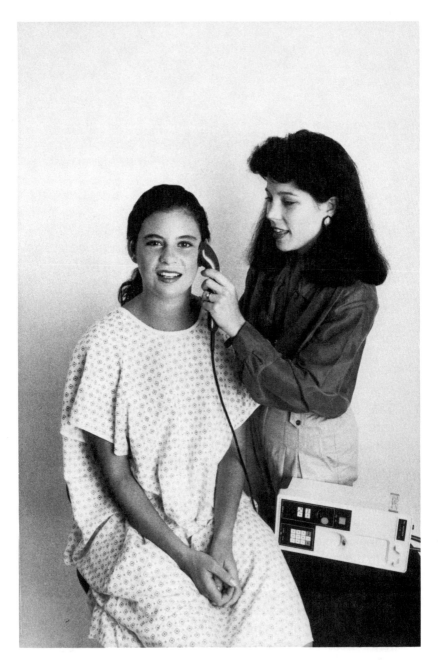

Ultrasound

of the muscles of your neck, back, and face. Your physical therapist will evaluate your cervical spine to determine if this is contributing to your TMJ problem, and may recommend referrals to either a neurologist or orthopedist.

Your physical therapist can teach you to do most of these techniques by yourself. After a series of visits to a physical therapist, you will probably be able to do most of the techniques at home. The education about your jaw muscles and joints can help you be much more comfortable. You may then need the help of a physical therapist only for flare-ups, such as times of stress or a re-injury to the joint.

What types of treatments will your physical therapist do?

1. Heat. Your physical therapist may use heat on your muscles and joints, which increases the blood flow to the area and allows for faster healing.

2. Ice. Cold reduces pain, swelling, and inflammation and allows the muscles and joints to increase their opening.

3. Ultrasound. Ultrasound is painless sound waves that are applied to your joint and muscles to reduce the pain and swelling and promote healing of the tissues.

4. Electrical stimulation. An electrical impulse is sent through your skin and causes your muscles to gently contract. This involuntary contraction stimulates the muscles and strengthens them, which decreases swelling and pain.

5. Jaw exercises. Exercises for your jaw muscles, like exercise for any muscles in your body, will help increase circulation and relax the muscles. It will also improve your flexibility and range of motion. Exercises help to heal the muscles and joints, increase the lubrication of the joints, and release chemicals into the blood, which can reduce pain. Jaw exercises can be as simple as standing in front

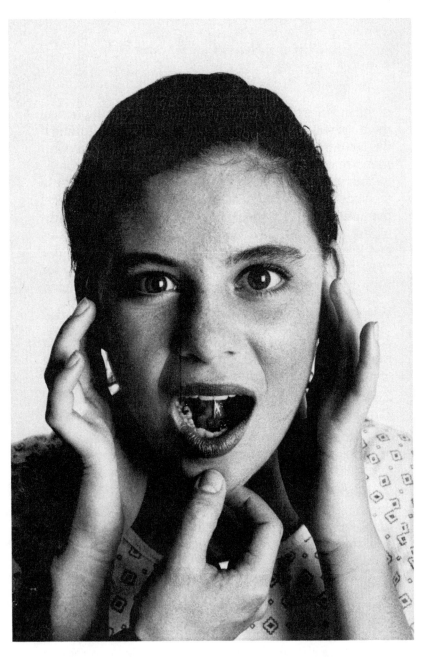

Physical Therapist Helping With Jaw Exercise

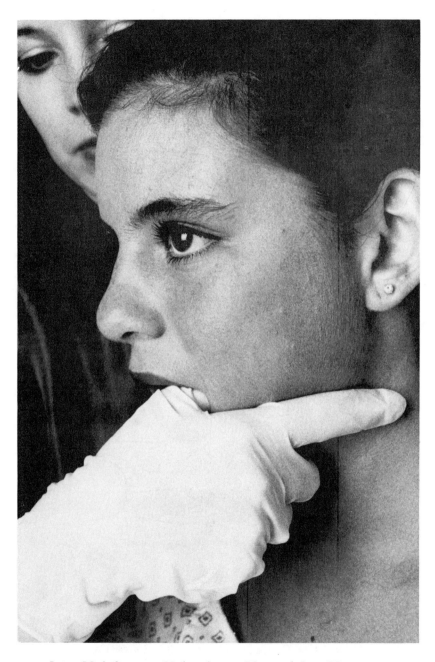

Joint Mobilization Helps Attain Normal Jaw Movement

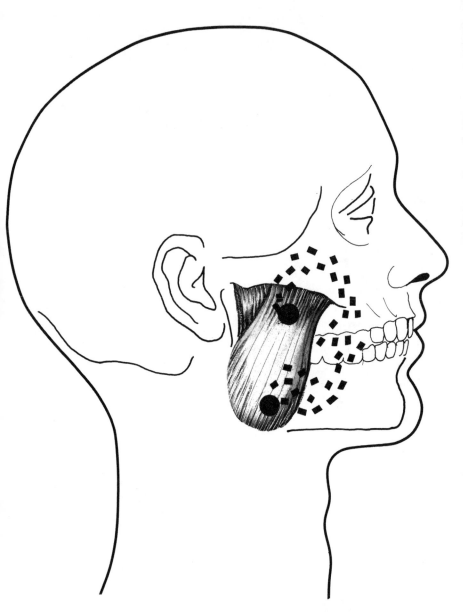

Referred Pain Patterns (■) From Painful Knots (•) In Masseter
Muscle Can Cause Pain To Be Felt In Distant Areas
Such As Teeth, Cheek, And Lower Jaw.

of a mirror and opening and closing your jaw in a straight line, or placing the tip of your tongue on the front part of your palate and making a click, click sound. There are many other exercises that may be recommended, depending on your particular problem.

6. Joint mobilization. Damaged joints and muscles often have a limited range of motion due to muscle spasm, muscle shortening, or adhesions in the joint itself. Your physical therapist will help you get the maximum amount of movement out of your jaw and, in doing this, help relieve the causes of restricted movement as well as promote healing and lubrication of the joint and muscles.

Another technique to increase the range of motion of your jaw is called spray and stretch. This is a technique whereby your physical therapist finds the trigger points in your muscles. These are points that are very tender to touch and that refer pain to areas away from the muscle. Stretching the muscle and directing cold spray along the bands of the muscle loosens up the muscle so that it can stretch farther and reduces the pain in the muscle trigger point.

7. Massage. Massage will help stimulate and heal your sore muscles. It will help identify the areas of muscles that are under tension or have knots or sore spots in them. It can also help identify areas of pain in your muscles that refer pain away from the muscle. This can be very important in educating you as to where the pain source is. Pain that is unknown can often cause anxiety, and simply being able locate the source of pain will help reduce anxiety about it. Massage also feels good and can reduce the pain in your muscles and joint and help you to see what it will feel like to be with less pain.

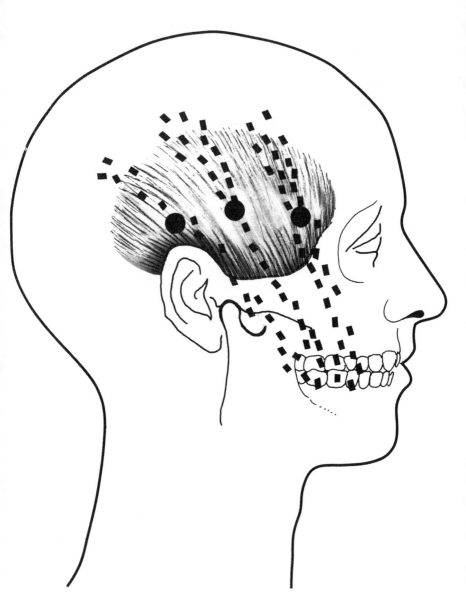

Referred Pain Patterns (■) From Painful Knots (●) In Temporalis
Muscle Can Cause Pain To Be Felt In Distant Areas
Such As Teeth, Forehead, And Temple Areas.

8. Education and prevention. Your physical therapist will teach you how to improve the posture of your head, neck, shoulders, and jaw. Physical therapists can also show you the relationship between tension and the way you hold yourself. They can show you how stress makes itself felt in specific parts of your body and how it feels to have your back, shoulders, neck, and jaw in a relaxed position. You will then be able to recognize when you are under stress and when parts of your body tense up. This is one of the most important lessons to learn in order to be able to overcome muscle tension and its often painful outcomes.

Chiropractic Treatment

Chiropractors provide much of the health care for people in the United States, especially for those with back problems and back pain. However, a large section of the medical community does not accept chiropractic treatment and some even claim that chiropractors' treatment of adjusting the spine can cause serious injury to the spinal cord. But the fact is that many people are helped by chiropractors.

Back problems are largely caused by muscle spasm, a problem that chiropractors are fairly skilled at dealing with. They emphasize stress reduction and relaxation as well as adjustment of the spine. They use other techniques such as massage, spray and stretch, heat, ice, and electrical stimulation of the muscles to improve symptoms of muscle pain. Many TMJ problems, especially TMJ muscle problems, are associated with tightness of muscles of the neck and even with tightness of muscles of the upper back. By relieving this muscle tension in the upper back and neck, many TMJ muscle problems are greatly improved.

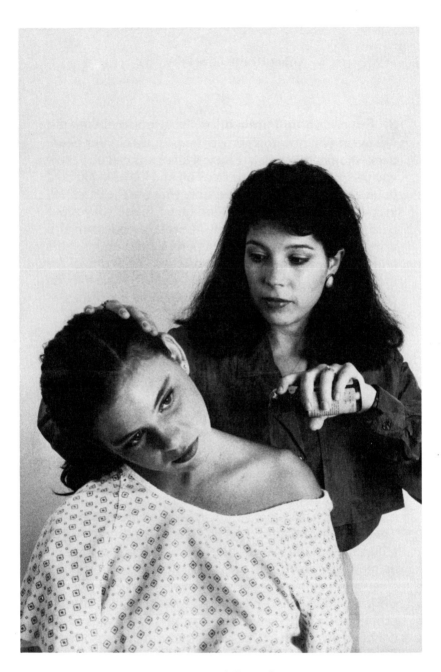

Spray And Stretch

In addition, chiropractors are experts in posture, a contributing factor in TMJ muscle problems. People who carry their head forward often have muscle tension in their neck and jaw muscles, and this needs to be corrected by improving their posture. I have had many patients who have been helped by chiropractors, many of whom use some of the same techniques as physical therapists.

A recent article noted that a dentist went back to school and got his chiropractic degree and started a clinic for TMJ patients at a dental school, utilizing both the insights of dentistry and chiropractic. It will be interesting to see what success this approach has for the treatment of TMJ problems.

Acupuncture

The Needles That Helped Diane

Diane had a history of headaches for the past few years. She was under a lot of stress in her job as a secretary and had to take time off work once or twice a month because of severe headaches. My examination showed that in addition to the grinding of her teeth and the stress that she exhibited, she also had soreness of her temporomandibular joints as well as the muscles in her cheek and temple areas. All the standard treatments such as physical therapy, pain medication, soft diet, exercises, heat and ice, and a splint did not do much to improve her condition. We decided to try acupuncture. After the first treatment, she felt that her headaches had gotten much better. After two more acupuncture treatments, she felt that her headaches had improved and were now 90 percent reduced.

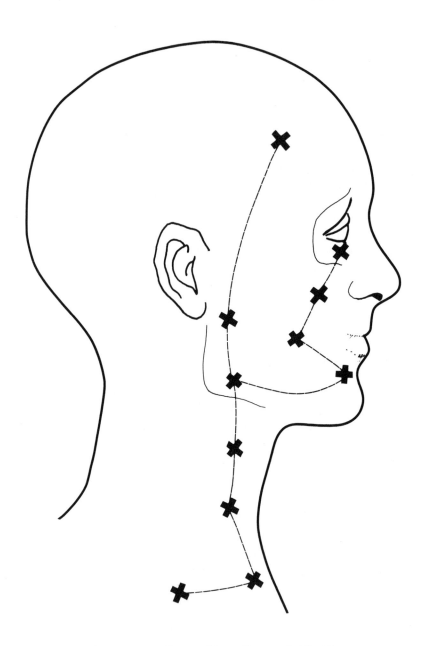

**Acupuncture Points Along Stomach Meridian
On Head And Neck**

Acupuncture is the insertion of needles into specific areas of the body that have been determined by ancient Chinese medicine. Western scientific theory cannot completely explain how acupuncture works, but it does work. Acupuncture can provide relief for many TMJ problems.

What do we know about how acupuncture works? One theory is that acupuncture stimulates the release of chemicals called endorphins — or naturally occurring pain-killers — into the bloodstream, which act as a drug to alleviate pain. Acupuncture also works as a type of anesthesia. It is used in China as anesthesia for many surgical procedures, including tooth extraction and surgery. How acupuncture causes anesthesia is not completely understood, however.

Some people believe that acupuncture works because people believe in acupuncture and that it will do what they believe. But studies have shown that this is not the case. When acupuncture treatments have been given to skeptical patients and to trusting patients, the best results have come from the skeptical patients. This is contrary to what one would expect if the effect of acupuncture was due to the patients' belief that it was going to work for them.

Often TMJ pain is caused by muscle spasm or sore spots, which then causes more pain, which causes more muscle spasm. Acupuncture can break the pain-muscle-spasm cycle and thus allows the structures then to heal.

Acupuncture also seems to have a relaxing and stress-relieving effect on patients. Anything that relaxes and lessens the stress is going to be beneficial for TMJ problems.

Acupuncture has been used quite successfully for the treatment of arthritis in other parts of the body and for muscle pain in the back. There has not been a lot of research on the use of acupuncture specifically for TMJ problems, but acupuncture's success in other parts of the body indicates it may also be successful for TMJ problems.

Acupuncture has to be kept in perspective: it is not a miracle cure. Having used acupuncture for the treatment of TMJ patients, I have found that it works on some patients and not on others. It should be regarded as one possible form of treatment, just like medication, which works better for some patients than for others.

Acupuncture has a cumulative effect. It usually does not work miraculously with one treatment. You need a series of treatments. Sometimes the symptoms will become worse immediately following the first treatment, but then they will subside and the symptoms will improve somewhat. The most improvement is felt after the completion of a series of treatments. Once the symptoms have improved, acupuncture is needed only when the symptoms start to reappear.

Counseling and Support Groups

Both individual counseling and support groups can help you manage stress and emotional feelings that have an effect upon your TMJ pain. Being able to talk to someone about these feelings can help you feel more in control of your emotions and therefore keep your emotions from controlling you.

TMJ problems can be due largely to somatization of emotions. In other words, we protect our hearts with shoulder and neck tension, and bite back anger with our jaw muscles. Many psychologists have talked about body armoring. These muscular habits of armoring, poor posture, and tension holding are intimately related to TMJ problems.

Therapy, either group or individual, may be necessary to work out emotional issues with others or to become emotionally expressive. We need to be able to say what hurts, or makes us angry or afraid. We need to become self-reliant, not excessively dependent on others. We need to learn to play more. We need to love our children, our family, and our partner. We need to slow down and enjoy life. We need to change how we function in society and this requires some sort of help or therapy.

Stress, as we have seen, plays a big role in TMJ problems. Individual or group support may help you learn how to manage stress. Knowing that other people have similar problems and seeing how they have managed their problems can also help.

If you have an especially stressful event in your life, individual or group support can often be helpful in bringing that event under control and not allowing it to have a harmful effect on your life.

Biofeedback

Biofeedback is the use of special equipment to measure the body's automatic responses. By observing these responses, you are then able to practice exerting control over them. Typically, you will have wires taped to your skin to measure muscle activity. The wires are connected to a measuring device that shows how much muscle tension you have. By practicing relaxation exercises, you can learn to control the amount of muscle tension. This is called biofeedback training.

Biofeedback training, when practiced regularly, can dramatically increase your ability to relax. This can noticeably reduce muscle tension, and inasmuch as muscle tension affects your TMJ problem, it can help in solving that problem. Many people express anxiety and frustration through muscle tension, which can irritate and injure both the muscles and the joint. Because biofeedback teaches recognition and control of that muscle tension, it can lead to improvement of TMJ problems.

Biofeedback seems to have an effect on control of muscle tension only during periods of consciousness. It is not very effective for bruxism, or grinding your teeth, and excess use of your jaw muscles during sleeping. There are biofeedback devices that can be worn at night, however. They sound an alarm whenever your muscles become tense and you start grinding your teeth. But these devices seem to work only as long as you are wearing them; once you remove them, you seem to go back to your same old habits.

Even though biofeedback can be helpful in many instances, it is not the answer to all TMJ problems. It is a form of relaxation, like yoga and meditation. Its main drawback is the cost. Biofeedback training can run from $500 to $1,000. For patients for whom other forms of relaxation, such as meditation and yoga are not practical, biofeedback may be very helpful. But biofeedback has to be practiced in conjunction with understanding stress in general. You need to be aware of how you react to stressful situations and the steps you can take to control the stress. Biofeedback is just one more technique that can help you control and change the negative affects of stress.

Stress management classes are a good source of learning how to manage stress. They are commonly given by community educational centers and hospitals.

Cranial Osteopathy

Cranial osteopathy involves manipulation of the bones of the skull. The theory is that the bones of the skull are able to move at the junction or sutures where they join. If these bones become misaligned, they can create an interference with the proper movement of spinal fluid. This type of manipulation has provided relief to many patients. The relief people experience is not yet completely understood.

This type of manipulation can be performed by many practitioners from osteopaths who are medically licensed with similar training to medical doctors, physical therapists, or other practitioners who have learned the method.

The Alexander Technique

The Alexander technique is an educational method of increasing your awareness of posture, balance, and movement. It is a way of moving more efficiently, in which a lighter, truer balance is found. One learns the relationship of the head, neck, and back so that there is less stress in the body.

It is an educational technique taught through manual guidance and verbal instruction. It is not a therapy, and teachers will tell you it may help your TMJ problem, but they make no promises. If it helps it would be a side benefit, but many people do find that problems with their back, neck, and TMJ are helped.

Teachers receive a certificate after three years of training, but there is nothing to stop others with very little training from teaching the Alexander technique.

The Feldenkrais Method

The Feldenkrais method is a learning method that can be of value to many patients. It teaches awareness through movement. It is done both in groups and individually. People are taught a series of movements of the head, neck, eyes, jaw, back and other parts of the body. The movements are done slowly, carefully, and gently, and some movements are quite complicated, such as moving your jaw and eyes together in the same direction and then in the opposite direction.

One usually needs eight to ten classes to learn the basic method. The method teaches you to be more aware of your body and tension. People find they are more relaxed, have better posture, and are more aware of the stress in their body.

Teachers should have a certificate that shows they have had three to six years of training. Unfortunately, anyone with very little training can call him or herself a Feldenkrais teacher.

CHAPTER 10

COSTS AND INSURANCE

It is hard to give an exact cost for any treatment because costs vary from provider to provider and from location to location, but even so there are some general estimates that will get you in the ballpark. Phase I treatment, or basic treatment to get you in a position where you can manage your TMJ problem, should cost less than $1,000 unless some expensive tests are ordered.

Below are some of the various costs:

1. Diagnosis . . . . $100 — 200
2. X-rays $200
3. MRI $800
4. Splint . . . . $400 — 1,000
5. Physical Therapy . . $50-100 per visit
   (usually 3-10 visits)
6. Medication . . . . $10-30 per week
7. Biofeedback . . . . . . $500 — 1,000

You can see that the estimate of $1,000 can be easily

exceeded depending on how serious your problem is and what you need. Often dental schools located in many large cities have TMJ clinics that can offer reduced rates.

Insurance

Insurance coverage has been historically a problem. Dentists have been in the forefront of the treatment for TMJ disorders. Many expensive dental procedures such as grinding the teeth so that they fit together better, placing caps on crowns on the teeth, or performing orthodontics have been recommended as a treatment for TMJ disorders. Therefore, in order to save money, most insurance companies have excluded any TMJ treatment from their dental policies. In addition, insurance companies did not want to be responsible for paying TMJ treatment on the teeth, so most medical insurance excludes any dental work. Thus, most TMJ treatment has been excluded from health insurance policies.

But today things are changing. There seems to be general agreement among both the medical and dental professions that TMJ disorders are medical problems, and should be covered by medical insurance, regardless of whether treated by a dentist or doctor. At present, ten states have laws, regulations or directions requiring health insurance policies issued within their state to include coverage for the diagnosis and treatment of temporomandibular joint disorders on the same basis as any other joint disorder.

In summary, many medical insurance policies cover TMJ treatment using the same basic therapies as are used for other joints. Diagnosis, X-rays, MRI, splints, physical therapy, medications, counseling and surgery are usually covered. But dental treatment is excluded.

This question still has to be further resolved, and lawsuits and patient pressure will help to make health insurance cover treatment of TMJ disorders. It seems unfair that one joint in the body can be excluded from insurance coverage.

More and more people get their health care through health maintenance organizations (HMOs). Very few of these have dental coverage, so doctors rather than dentists are usually the ones involved in the treatment. Often the care is not as good as it could be if it were performed by someone with more specialization, but some HMOs refer problem cases to specialists.

Sample Patient Letter To Insurance Company

The Insurance Company
P.O. Box 30992
Salt Lake City, UT 84130

Re: Jane Doe
       Plan #
       Rejection of Claim filed by:

Dear

I have been notified that the claim filed on my policy for services rendered by the above named dentist has been denied (copy of denial enclosed). Please be informed that I did not seek this therapy for a dental problem (as indicated by the I.C.D.A. codes on the claim form). I was referred to this dentist for diagnosis and treatment of the head, neck, face and temporomandibular joint symptoms that I experienced.

As my insurance carrier, I know you must realize that

the insurance code for this state does not allow denial of benefits to an insured on the basis of the type of health care license held by the practitioner.

If there is a clause in my policy where the service on the rejected claim is specifically excluded, please provide me with a copy of this specific language. If you cannot, I expect prompt payment of this claim.

I would appreciate your immediate attention in this matter. If this cannot be resolved, I will be forced to seek arbitration through my state insurance commission and/or refund of my health care premiums.

Sincerely,

cc: Dentist
    State Insurance Commission

CHAPTER 11
PREVENTION OF TMJ PROBLEMS

We all know that the best cure is prevention. Prevention in many areas of health has to do with controlling behavior. Heart disease can in part be prevented by good diet and exercise. Cancer risk can be lowered by not smoking. TMJ disorders can be prevented in many cases, and the risk can certainly be lowered. Below are some areas of importance.

1. **Take care of your body.** A healthy body functions better and stays healthy. Your teeth and gums are also very important for the stability of your TMJ and facial muscles. Good oral hygiene and care of your mouth can help you to keep your teeth for a lifetime.

2. **Follow a healthy diet.** Eat less fat, especially those fats contained in red meat. Eat more fish and seafood; they contain fats that are beneficial to your health. Eat fresh fruits and vegetables, especially those in season.

Eat lots of whole grains. Avoid highly refined flour and sugar. Avoid alcohol, caffeine, and tobacco. A healthy diet will make your whole body feel better as well as have a beneficial effect on your mind.

3. **Regular exercise** is also necessary for the proper functioning of your body and mind. Find a way to exercise at least four times a week for a minimum of 30 minutes. Do something that you enjoy such as dancing, bicycling, or swimming. Even walking can be beneficial — walk to work, walk to the store. Try not to use mechanical transportation whenever you can walk. Some people can build exercise into their regular lives by walking, and walking up stairs instead of taking elevators. You would be surprised to see how much of modern life deters us from exercise — elevators, escalators, cars, buses, taxis, etc.

4. **Control of distress** is very important in preventing muscle tightness and grinding of teeth. Distress is also very unhealthy generally, and is a contributing factor in ulcers, heart disease, cancer, and mental health. Recognizing stress and taking steps to cope with it is important. Relaxation techniques, individual or group support, and exercise can all help you reduce stress in your life.

5. **Physical injury** is a significant cause of TMJ disorders and much of it can be prevented. Automobile accidents are common and can be prevented by driving carefully and defensively. Wear seat belts and have headrests. Air bags hopefully will be available in the near future. Don't drink and drive.

   Contact sports are also a source of TMJ injuries. Wear a mouthpiece when playing contact sports such as football, basketball, hockey, boxing and rugby.

Another significant course of TMJ injuries is violence. Fighting, whether between unrelated individuals or spouses and other family members, is very often related to the abuse of drugs and alcohol. Help should be sought out for drug and alcohol problems.

Notes

GLOSSARY

Acupuncture — an ancient Chinese method of medical treatment based on placing needles in various points of the body.

Acupressure — A type of massage that utilizes the same points of the body as acupuncture.

Analgesia — The relief of pain. Usually provided by medications known as "pain killers."

Anesthesia — Putting a part of the body to sleep (local anesthesia) or the whole person to sleep (general anesthesia).

Arthritis — Inflammation of a joint. A class of diseases that cause inflammation of joints.

Arthroscopic surgery — A technique of surgery using small tubes inserted into a joint. One tube provides the light and a camera that shows the joint on a screen. Another tube is used to insert small surgical instruments, and repair the joint.

Biofeedback — The training that enables a person to control the body's automatic responses. Used to enhance relaxation and reduction of stress.

Bruxism — The grinding of teeth that is done while sleeping. Can cause wear to teeth and soreness to the jaw muscles and joints.

Chiropractor — A health practitioner whose expertise is adjusting and manipulating the spinal column.

Cranio-mandibular joint — The joint where the lower jaw or mandible attaches to the cranium or skull. Also known as the temporomandibular joints or TMJs.

Herbs — Plants that are used for their medicinal properties.

Ligament — Tough, fibrous tissue connecting two or more bones or cartilages.

Magnetic Resonance Imaging — Also known as MRI. A technique of magnetizing a part of the body and then passing sound waves through it to produce and image that is good for seeing soft tissues.

Malocclusion — A bad bite. Teeth that do not properly fit together.

Micro-Trauma — Small traumatic episodes such as those caused by grinding and clenching teeth that can cause damage over a long period of time.

Migraine Headache — A type of vascular headache characterized by pain on one side of the head, nausea, and visual disturbances.

Minerals — Naturally occurring inorganic chemicals that are necessary for the human diet.

Myofascial Pain — Trigger points that are small, painful knots located in various muscles of the body that produce referred pain.

Myositis — Inflammation of a muscle usually causing pain.

NSAID — Non-steroidal, anti-inflammatory drugs. A class of drugs that reduces inflammation. May also relieve pain.

Orthognathic Surgery — A surgery to reposition the jaw bones.

Orthotic — Also known as a splint. Usually a plastic appliance that fits over the teeth and repositions the jaw.

Physical Therapy — The treatment of disease by mechanical means such as heat, cold, light, and massage.

Referred Pain — Pain that is felt in a part of the body distant from where the source of the pain is located.

Sinusitis — Inflammation of the lining of the sinus, which often causes a headache.

Synovial Fluid — The lubricating fluid that is present in joints and responsible for the smooth movement.

Tinnitus — A ringing in the ears.

Ultrasound — A treatment using sound waves that can't be heard to help heal injured tissues.

Vitamins — Organic naturally occurring chemicals that are necessary for human metabolism.

Whiplash — An injury where the neck is bent backwards and then forwards. It often causes injuries to the jaw muscles and joints.

Author's Note

Readers' comments or suggestions are welcomed. I hope to update this book periodically and would like to answer any questions readers may have. I can be reached through the publisher, Aurora Press, P.O. Box 573, Santa Fe, NM 87504.

Below are listed two organizations that can refer readers to specialists in the TMJ Field:

**American Academy of Head, Neck,
Facial Pain and TMJ Orthopedics
613 West Cedar Street
Hurst, TX 76053
Tel: 800-322-8651**

**American Academy of
Craniomandibular Disorders
10 Joplin Ct.
Layfayette, CA 94549**

APPENDIX

SUGGESTED FOODS FOR SOFT FOOD DIET

FOODS TO EAT	FOODS TO AVOID

Dairy

milk, whole or skimmed, yogurt, sour cream, cottage cheese, all cheeses when cooked or melted, eggs, scrambled, soft, boiled, poached, butter, margarine

hard cheeses, fried or hard boiled eggs

Bread

breads with crust removed if soaked until soft, or soft in a cooked dish, soft pancakes or French toast without crust, cooked cereals: oatmeal, Farina, Cream of Wheat, Cream of Rice, corn meal mush

granola, dry cereals, nuts or raisins in cereals

Vegetables

pureed vegetables, well cooked, soft vegetables, mashed potatoes, baked potatoes removed from skin and mashed, sweet potatoes removed from skin, creamed spinach or broccoli, beans cooked until very soft or mashed, refried beans, creamed corn

raw vegetables, carrots, celery, lettuce, potato chips, fried rice

Fruits

cooked apples or pears, applesauce, soft ripe bananas, juices and nectars, orange juice, grapefruit juice, apricot nectar, any fruit run through a blender

raw fruits, dried fruits

Soups

split pea, bean, potato, lentil, leek, chicken noodles, beef broth, onion

any hard or chewable pieces of meat or vegetable, clams

Pasta

any well cooked pasta such as spaghetti, noodles, vermicelli, linguine, etc., sauces without chewable pieces

clam sauce, meat sauce

Casseroles

macaroni and cheese, tuna casserole, eggplant casserole, potato casserole, squash casserole

meat, stringy or hard vegetables

Meats

meats and fish can be put in blender and pureed, canned tuna or salmon can be used in casseroles, meat stews can be blended into thick soups

all meats that require chewing

Desserts

ice cream without fruit or nuts, sherbert, yogurt, custard, Jello, puddings, tapioca, milk shakes, fruit drinks run through blender

candy, nuts, fruit

SAMPLE SOFT FOOD DIET

1. Breakfast
   Grapefruit juice, soft boiled egg, cream of wheat with milk, stewed prunes, decaf coffee or tea with milk

   Mid-morning
   Eggnog with orange juice

   Lunch
   Cream of onion soup, macaroni and cheese casserole, sherbert

   Snack
   Custard

   Dinner
   Cream of mushroom or split pea soup, potato (mashed or baked and removed from skin) with butter, creamed tuna on well cooked noodles, Jello with banana

2. Breakfast
   orange juice, scrambled egg, soft pancake with butter and syrup, decaf coffee or tea with milk

   Mid-morning
   blended drink of milk and canned peaches

   Lunch
   cottage cheese with applesauce, beef stew put through blender, ice cream

   Snack
   Yogurt

   Dinner
   chicken noodle soup, spaghetti with mushroom sauce, creamed spinach, chocolate pudding

---

Helpful Hint: A blender and juicer are very handy for soft diets. Almost any meal can be put through a blender (e.g., meat, fish, vegetables) and can be eaten without chewing. The same is true for most fruits and vegetables; they can be made into healthy, nutritious juices such as carrot, apple, or tomato. Use your imagination. V-8 is made of eight different vegetables. Delicious shakes can be made with fruits blended with milk, yogurt or juices. Banana and pineapple, peaches or strawberries with milk, and pineapple with coconut milk are some examples.

QUIZ — True or False
(Answers on next page)

1. THE CHEWING MUSCLES PLAY AN IMPORTANT ROLE IN THE FUNCTIONING OF THE TMJ.   T F

2. MOST HEADACHES ARE CAUSED BY SOMETHING BEING WRONG WITH THE TMJ.   T F

3. EARACHES CAN BE CAUSED BY A DISORDER OF THE TMJ.   T F

4. CAR ACCIDENTS CAN CAUSE TMJ PROBLEMS.   T F

5. YOU NEED AN X-RAY TO DIAGNOSE A TMJ PROBLEM.   T F

6. GRINDING YOUR TEETH (BRUXISM) WILL ALWAYS CAUSE TMJ PROBLEMS.   T F

7. STRESS IS VERY IMPORTANT IN TMJ DISORDERS.   T F

8. DENTAL TREATMENT IS IMPORTANT TO STOP TMJ PAIN.   T F

9. TMJ DISORDERS THAT ARE STILL PAINFUL AFTER SIX MONTHS OF TREATMENT WILL REQUIRE SURGERY.   T F

10. MOST TMJ PROBLEMS CAN BE TOTALLY CURED.   T F

Answers To Quiz

1. **True.** There are four main jaw muscles that open and close the mouth.
2. **False.** Even though a disorder of the TMJ can cause headaches, most headaches are from other causes.
3. **True.** Pain can be referred from the TMJ to the ear.
4. **True.** Car accidents that involve a direct blow to the jaw or a whiplash can cause injury to both the TMJ and/or the face and neck muscles.
5. **False.** Many TMJ disorders can be diagnosed without an x-ray, but your doctor may want an x-ray to help diagnose some types of TMJ disorders.
6. **False.** Grinding your teeth will often cause sore muscles and sore jaw joints, but most people grind their teeth to some extent with little or no TMJ problems.
7. **True.** Stress is important to control because it is related to muscle tension and grinding the teeth. Stress is also important in controlling pain.
8. **False.** Dental treatment may be important for a healthy, well functioning, and nice looking mouth, but TMJ pain should be controlled before having dental work, and you should understand that dental work will probably have very little affect on your TMJ pain.
9. **False.** Only a small percentage of TMJ disorders require surgery, even when there is pain after six months. There needs to be a problem that can be corrected by surgery.
10. **False.** Most TMJ problems can be managed so that you can live a happy, normal life. But you must recognize you have a weakness and try to prevent problems from starting, and learn how to care for any problem that does arise when it first starts so that you do not have serious recurrences.

SUGGESTED READINGS

Benson, Herbert, M.D. *The Relaxation Response.*
William Morrow & Company, 1975.

Boston Women's Health Collective, Inc. *Our Bodies,
Ourselves.* Simon And Schuster, 1976.

Boyd, Doug. *Rolling Thunder.* Dell Publishing Co.,
Inc., 1974.

Chaitow, Leon, N.D.O.O. *Instant Pain Control.*
Thorsons Publishing Group, England, 1984.

Cooper, Kenneth H. *The Aerobics Way.* J. Evans And
Co., 1977.

Cousins, Norman. *Anatomy of an Illness.* Bantam
Books, Inc., 1983.

Davis, Adele. *Lets Eat Right to Keep Fit.* Harcourt,
Brace, Janovich, Inc., 1954.

Dickson, Murray. *Where There is No Dentist.*
Hesperian Foundation, 1983.

Downing, George. *The Massage Book.* Random
House, 1972.

Hittleman, Richard. *Richard Hittleman's 30 Day Yoga
Meditation Plan.* Bantam Books, Inc., 1978.

McNeill, Charles, DDS (Ed). *Craniomandibular
Disorders Guidelines for Evaluation, Diagnosis, and
Management; The Academy of Craniomandibular
Disorders,* Quintessence Publishing Co, Inc. 1991.

Pritikin, Nathan. *The Pritikin Program for Diet and
Exercise.* Grosset and Dunlap, 1979.

Saper, Joel, R.M.D. and Magee, Kenneth, M.D.
Freedom from Headaches. Simon and Schuster,
1981.

Shealy, Norman. 90 Days to Self Health. Dial Press,
1977.

Samuels, Mike, M.D. and Bennet, Hal. *The Well Body Book*. Random House, 1973.

Travell, Janet, M.D. and Simons, David G. *Myofascial Pain and Dysfunction: The Trigger Point Manual*. Williams and Wilkins, 1983.

Ward, Matthew. *Seven Herbs, Plants as Teachers*. North Atlantic Books, 1987.

Weiner, Michael A. *Earth Medicine — Earth Foods*. MacMillan Publishing Co., 1972.

Wilson, Randy. *The Non-Chew Cook Book*. Wilson Publishing, Box 2190, Glenwood Springs, Colorado, 816702.

Notes

INDEX

171

Index

ABOUT THE AUTHOR

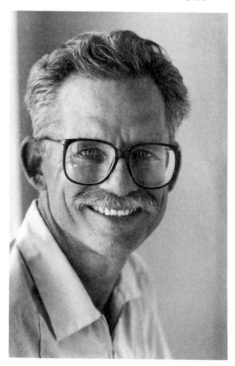

Dr. Greg Goddard attended the University of California Medical Center at San Francisco, becoming a Doctor of Dental Surgery in 1967. He did his Oral Surgery Residency at Royal Free Hospital in London, England, where he studied and practiced the treatment of temporomandibular joint and muscle problems, using the methods that orthopedic surgeons use to treat other joints. Since 1975 Dr. Goddard has been licensed in California to practice acupuncture for the treatment of dental and facial pain.

Dr. Goddard is currently Dental Director of the Native American Health Center in San Francisco. This clinic provides care for Native American Indian patients in the San Francisco Bay Area. Hundreds of these patients have been treated by Dr. Goddard for various types of pain and disorders of the temporomandibular joints.

Other Titles From Aurora

COMING HOME

A Guide to Dying at Home With Dignity
Deborah Duda

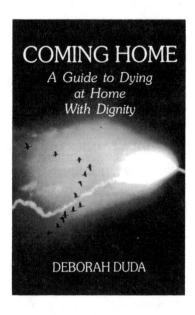

"This is a superb encyclopedia of information on a process which was the rule until our most recent generation. Perhaps the most important aspects of the book are the discussion of when it is not appropriate to die at home (not very often but primarily when the family and patient don't want it to happen!). For those persons who are really turned off by the problem of dying in a hospital and who don't have medical expertise to make many of the decisions on their own, this is a book worth reading. It includes the dying person's bill of rights, originally created by the Southwestern Michigan Inservice Education Council. In an age of social transformation where financial resources alone may lead to more individuals choosing to die at home, this is a worthwhile guide for lay persons and can be confidently recommended by health care professionals for those individuals seeking such information."

C. NORMAN SHEALY, M.D., Ph.D.

THE EAR: GATEWAY TO BALANCING THE BODY

A MODERN GUIDE TO EAR ACUPUNCTURE

Mario Wexu, D.AC

This is the first comprehensive modern textbook of ear acupuncture. The author uniquely combines his extensive personal clinical experience with traditional and modern Chinese and European sources. Anatomical descriptions with detailed charts clearly illustrate how to locate and use over three hundred ear points, both alone and in combination with body points, to treat and prevent illness. Case histories with specific techniques cover problems such as:

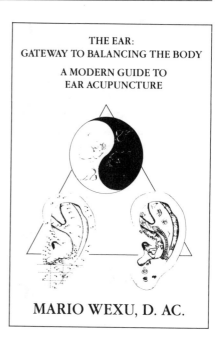

THE EAR:
GATEWAY TO BALANCING THE BODY

A MODERN GUIDE TO
EAR ACUPUNCTURE

MARIO WEXU, D. AC.

- Deafness
- Otitis
- Otalgia
- Drug Addiction
- Tobacco Addiction
- Alcoholism

- Obesity
- Anesthesia
- Oedema
- Insomnia
- Acupuncture Anesthesia
- Electronic Acupuncture Devices

An incredible repertory listing 130 diseases facilitates an understanding of this incredible and valuable healing art.

SILVER DENTAL FILLINGS THE TOXIC TIMEBOMB

Can The Mercury In Your Dental Fillings Poison You?

Sam Ziff

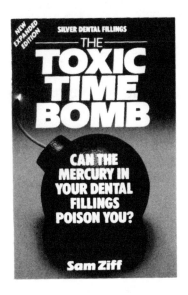

A significant and shocking expose of one of the greatest health dangers of our time. The amalgam used to fill teeth is 40 to 50 per cent mercury, a known poison. This book explains how mercury migrates from the teeth into the body affecting our overall health in a dramatic manner. This groundbreaking book includes the following topics and questions:

• Mercury in Medicine and Dentistry • The History of Mercury in Medicine • The Arguments For and Against • Do we really have electricity in our mouths? • Measurement of Mercury in the urine • How long does it stay in the body? • Mercury in the body, where does it go? • Does Mercury cause any changes in our tissues and organs? • Does Mercury cause psychiatric and behavioral changes? • Micromercurialism, signs and symptoms

This pioneering book is written in a clear straightforward manner, ideal for the layman and professional who want to become aware of the body of information currently available on mercury toxicity from dental amalgams. Then, informed, each individual can draw his own conclusions.

> "Silver Dental Fillings *alerts the reader to the need for more research and understanding of the role that mercury amalgam may have on chronic health dysfunction."* **JEFFREY BLAND, Ph.D.**